AI in Orthopedic Trauma Care 1

AI in Orthopedic Trauma Care 1

Comparative Clinical Insights

Edited by

Abhishek Kumar
Priya Batta

iSTE

WILEY

First published 2026 in Great Britain and the United States by ISTE Ltd and John Wiley & Sons, Inc.

ISTE Ltd
27-37 St George's Road
London SW19 4EU
UK

www.iste.co.uk

John Wiley & Sons, Inc.
111 River Street
Hoboken, NJ 07030
USA

www.wiley.com

Library of Congress Control Number: 2026936292

British Library Cataloguing-in-Publication Data
A CIP record for this book is available from the British Library
ISBN 978-1-83669-124-2

The manufacturer's authorized representative according to the EU General Product Safety Regulation is Wiley-VCH GmbH, Boschstr. 12, 69469 Weinheim, Germany, e-mail: Product_Safety@wiley.com.

Contents

Preface

This book explores how artificial intelligence (AI) is transforming the assessment, management and recovery of musculoskeletal injuries. By integrating machine learning (ML), deep learning (DL) and predictive analytics with advanced imaging and electronic health records (EHR), AI enhances fracture detection, risk stratification and personalized treatment planning. Data-driven models support clinicians in making accurate, timely decisions while optimizing rehabilitation pathways based on patient-specific factors. Continuous monitoring through wearable sensors further enables real-time feedback and adaptive recovery programs.

This book highlights how AI improves clinical efficiency, reduces complications and enhances functional outcomes. It also addresses ethical considerations, data governance and implementation challenges, offering a comprehensive perspective on the future of intelligent, precision-driven orthopedic trauma care systems.

Abhishek KUMAR
Priya BATTA
May 2026

1

AI-Assisted Comparison of Volar Plating with and Without Carpal Tunnel Release in Distal Radius Fractures

Volar plating is a common treatment method used to treat distal end radius fractures that are remedied with an open reduction and internal fixation (ORIF). Still, dysfunction of the median nerve that occurs after the operation and acute carpal tunnel syndrome (CTS) are also critical complications that might interfere with normal functioning. There are some controversies concerning the advantages of carrying out a prophylactic carpal tunnel release (CTR) during the fracture fixing.

This chapter provides an AI-aided comparison of the equivalent number of patients with uncomplicated distal radius fractures receiving volar plating with or without comorbid CTR. The emphasis is put on family outcomes, nerve conduction and functional recovery. The prospective recording of adult patients was performed. Follow-ups that were evaluated included a standardized clinical examination, nerve conduction studies (NCV/EMG), and Patient-Rated Wrist Evaluation (PRWE) scores assessed at predetermined intervals. The comparison of the incidence of CTS, severity of median nerve dysfunction, complication rates, and fracture union, as well as functional outcomes between the two groups, was carried out using an AI-assisted data analysis.

The results indicated that patients who received volar plating with concomitant CTR experienced remarkably reduced cases of ongoing symptoms of CTS, enhanced electrophysiological conditions and enhanced segregation outcomes, compared to those who obtained volar plating. Significantly, CTR was not associated with the increase in surgical complications or fracture healing. These results indicate that AI-based assessment enhances clinical judgment and that prophylactic CTR could be beneficially used by high-risk patients undergoing volar plating of a distal radius fracture.

Chapter written by Abhishek SHARMA and Paresh V. PATIL.

For a color version of all the figures in this chapter, see www.iste.co.uk/kumar/orthopedic1.zip.

1.1. Introduction

Fractures of the distal radius end are among the most frequent injuries in orthopedic practice and form much of the upper-limb global fractures (Ochen et al. 2020). They occur across all ages. The predominant reasons behind high-energy trauma include road traffic injury, sporting injury and injury on an outstretched hand, but low-energy injuries are more common among aged osteoporotic patients. Since the wrist articulation, transmission of loads and functions of the hand depend on the distal radius; anatomy is better managed by ensuring the maintenance of the motion and prevention of long-term disability (Buijze et al. 2021).

There has been a radical transformation in treatment patterns of the distal radius fractures in recent decades. The closed reduction and casting are still appropriate to stable fractures, but unstable, displaced and intra-articular ones could require surgical intervention to attain acceptable results (Coon et al. 2022).

The surgical technique that has best emerged is open reduction and internal fixation (ORIF) by using volar locking plates, since they provide biomechanical stability, anatomical reduction and early mobility of the wrist. Volar plating has demonstrated positive outcomes in both the young and elderly patients, and has replaced, in most cases, the use of dorsal plating and the use of long-term external fixation (Maccagnano et al. 2021).

Although these are advantages, volar plating may still produce complications. Irritation or rupture of tendons, pain consisting of implants, loss of reduction, infection and neurovascular problems have been reported (Kew and Brockmeier 2021). Of the latter, the compression of the median nerve resulting in CTS is of high relevance since it may acutely affect recovery after surgery.

CTS is a condition that occurs as the result of compression of the median nerve in the carpal tunnel, which brings about pain, numbness, tingling and hand-weakness. In distal radius fractures, CTS can either happen acutely due to displacement and swelling of the fracture or occur postoperatively due to plate irritation, fibrosis, changed biomechanics of the carpal tunnel or edema (Malakootian et al. 2023).

Postoperative CTS is hard to diagnose and treat. The early symptoms of the disease may be disguised by the pain and swelling and delay the diagnosis and therefore increase the chance of irreversible nerve loss (Pergolizzi et al. 2023). Acute CTS qualifies as an orthopedic emergency since when compression is prolonged, sensory and motor losses are irreversible. The objective measure of the median nerve functioning is the nerve conduction test (NCV) and electromyography (EMG), which ultimately gives a positive diagnosis of the condition, severity and progress (Reimann and Wijesekera 2022).

One of the main controversies about distal radius fracture management is the use of CTR as a prophylaxis in volar plating. The supporters base their argument on the fact that early decompression will help to prevent postoperative median nerve compression, decrease chronic CTS and provide better outcomes. Critics respond with the argument that routine CTR can be avoided since post-surgery CTS can be a temporary condition and can clear up with conservative treatment, and further surgery can be very debilitating (Barnes et al. 2021).

New technologies in artificial intelligence (AI) and analytics based on data provide new solutions to the dilemma. AI-assisted analysis has the potential to combine large sets of data containing demographic information, clinical results, electrophysiological and functional outcome scores (Williams 2024).

AI tools make the process of comparative evaluation of outcomes more objective and precise by identifying increasingly intricate patterns and forecasting values. AI has shown promise in the classification of fractures, prediction of outcomes and risk stratification of complication, although little has been done in terms of assessing nerve-related prognosis, even after fractures of the distal radius have been fixed.

A deeper assessment of volar plating can be performed through the use of AI-controlled analysis to compare the volar plating with or without CTR to highlight the slight changes of nerve conduction and functional recovery patterns that cannot be easily identified with conventional statistics. The method is beneficial, as it is capable of recognizing patients that are at high risk of undergoing surgery early, as well as assisting in the evidence-based decision-making process of surgery.

Functional recovery is one of the major objectives in the treatment of distal radius fracture. Patient-Rated Wrist Evaluation scores (PRWE) specifically, patient-reported measures, help us to understand the perspective of the patient on the level of pain, disability, and general functionality of the wrist. The PRWE scores can be added to the electrophysiological data to offer a complete evaluation of the objective nerve recovery and see functional improvement as subjective (John et al. 2022).

The current study will focus on making an AI-aided comparison of volar plating in comparison to not including concomitant carpal tunnel release (CTR) among patients with distal radius fractures. The data objectives include describing changes in nerve conduction after surgery, assessing the incidence and predictive variables of acute CTS and comparing the functional result and level of complication in the two forms of surgery. The proposed study aims to elucidate the value of prophylactic CTR and add some evidence to improving surgical management measures of distal radius fractures in order to optimize AI-based analysis of clinical, electrophysiological and functional data.

1.2. Literature review

The fractures at the distal radius are frequent and comprise 15–20% of all fractures (Mehta et al. 2024). They are represented in two ages: one group through high-energy injuries such as motorbike accidents, and older adults because of osteoporosis, which makes them fall when standing due to height. The objectives of treatment are straightforward; position the bone in absolute mode, make the fracture non-inflammatory and restore the function of the wrist and hand as soon as possible.

Conventionally, these fractures were treated by physicians using closed reduction and a cast. Malunion, stiffness and disillusioning functioning were, however, caused by unstable patterns. They altered the game when volar locking plates were released. These provide high fixation, particularly in weak bone. Many studies have verified that volar plates have superior alignment on X-ray, permit remobilization sooner and have a higher functional score than dorsal plates or external fixation (Laohaprasitiporn et al. 2022).

The most common compressive neuropathy of the upper limb is carpal tunnel syndrome (CTS). This is caused by the compression of the median nerve within a carpal tunnel. Patients experience numbness, weakness, tingling and pain along the median-nerve territory. Idiopathic CTS is well known; however, CTS after a distal radiate fracture has its own issues. It is increased by traumatic swellings, changed mechanics in the wrist and surgical predispositions (Lacinski et al. 2024).

It is well observed by many authors that a new CTS may be formed once a distal radius fracture has occurred. Carpal tunnel pressure is increased by swelling, blood clots or a displaced fracture. There is a great disparity in the rates reported (3–25%). Due to the possible permanent damage, the nerve may suffer due to long-term compression; the acute CTS is an emergency needing to be addressed within a short period of time.

Volar plating also excels regarding fracture stability, which may lead to median nerve issues following surgery. The problem has been associated by researchers with the position of plates that are positioned outside of the watershed line, excessive distal screws, agitated soft tissues and extended tourniquet periods. Fibrosis of the tunnel and scar tissue and enlarged synovium following surgery may also result in the squeeze of the nerve.

The surgery performed on a CTR cuts through the transverse carpal ligament to relieve pressure on the median nerve. The idiopathic CTS is the standard of CTR to use, but its proactive application during the repair of a distal radius fracture is debated.

Certain research believes that postoperative CTR reduces symptoms and improves functions in CTS prophylaxis, particularly in high-risk individuals. Others suggest that mild cases may clear themselves, so a wait-and-watch strategy is beneficial.

The gold standards of CTS diagnosis and the assessment of the degree of deceit involve NCV and EMG. Research has revealed that the delay in motor latency and slower sensory conductance is present among patients who develop CTS after a fracture. When these tests are used, an objective method is availed toward tracking nerve recovery in post-surgery patients (Hassan et al. 2021).

The PRWE is a typical patient-reported instrument to track pain and disability in the post-fracture of the distal radius (Hall et al. 2021; Kumar et al. 2026). It is consistently demonstrated in the results that patients in whom the median nerve compression is not treated, fair poorly. Premature nerve release results in faster recuperation, firm grip and an improved level of patient satisfaction.

Even though numerous studies are present, not many prospective comparisons have been performed concerning the shift in nerve conduction and functional outcomes between volar plating with CTR and without. Recent literature is exploring AI-based risk models and improvements and analysis that identify more at-risk patients in the process of postoperative CTS, which might be used to influence surgical decisions.

1.3. Materials and methods

1.3.1. *Study setting and ethical approval*

Our prospective study was conducted at the Orthopedics Department, KIMSDU, Karad, India. The Institutional Review Board endorsed it, and informed consent was obtained by the participants after full disclosure. The total duration of study was eighteen months.

1.3.2. *Study population and sample size*

A total of 34 patients diagnosed with distal end radius fractures and meeting the inclusion and exclusion criteria were enrolled in this prospective study. These patients were randomly distributed between two groups, with 17 patients in each group, to reduce selection bias and ensure comparability.

In total, 34 patients with inclusion criteria were studied from March 2023 to September 2024 (18 months):

n = 4pq/L2 p = Proportion of CTS in DER (14) q = 100-p
(100-14=86)
L = Precision = 12% n = 4 * 14 * 86/ 144 = 34

The sample size comes out to be 34.

– *Group 1*: 17 patients were treated with ORIF along with CTR in the course of surgery.

– *Group 2*: 17 patients were treated with ORIF without CTR.

We also calculated the size of the sample on previous studies and what would be feasible within the period of 18 months between March 2023 and September 2024.

We got 34 patients in an attempt to closely monitor and ensure our data met the standard of accuracy and compared before and after surgery the frequency of the CTS occurrence and subsequent functioning.

1.3.3. *Inclusion criteria*

– Age should be greater than eighteen years old.

– All types of distal end radius fractures.

– Radiographic/computed tomography (CT) scan confirmation of distal end radius fracture.

– Treated definitively with volar plating fixation.

1.3.4. *Exclusion criteria*

– Other tunnel syndromes: Guyon's canal, cubital tunnel, radial tunnel syndrome.

– Pre-existing CTS symptoms.

– Previous median nerve symptoms or prior CTR.

– Alcohol or drug abuse.

– Hematological disorders: hemophilia, thalassemia.

– Corticosteroid use.

– Prior upper limb surgeries.

– Osteoporosis or post-menopausal CTS-like symptoms.

– Age is less than eighteen years old.

– Non-adherence to follow-up protocol (six months).

– Thyroid disorders.

– Old fractures (greater than three weeks).

– History of compartment syndrome.

– Open fractures.

– Systemic diseases affecting nerve function or healing (e.g. diabetes mellitus, rheumatoid arthritis).

– Treatment strategies excluding volar plating.

1.3.5. *Study Groups*

The population of the study was separated into two groups:

– *Group 1*: ORIF with CTR as one operation.

– *Group 2*: ORIF without CTR.

1.3.6. *Preoperative assessment*

– History and clinical examination.

– X-ray: AP and lateral views of the wrist.

– EMG/NCV study for nerve conduction assessment (baseline).

– Application of the below-elbow slab under traction.

1.3.7. *Trauma-surgery interval*

Patients were given medications and elevation for three to four days prior to surgery to reduce swelling.

1.3.8. *Observation and result*

This study compared two surgical approaches for distal radius fractures with suspected carpal tunnel involvement:

– *Group A (ORIF + CTR)*: patients underwent ORIF with simultaneous CTR during the same surgical procedure. This combined approach addresses both the fracture and potential median nerve compression concurrently.

– *Group B (ORIF Alone)*: ORIF without CTR, in which case, it was not carried out when it was not indicated.

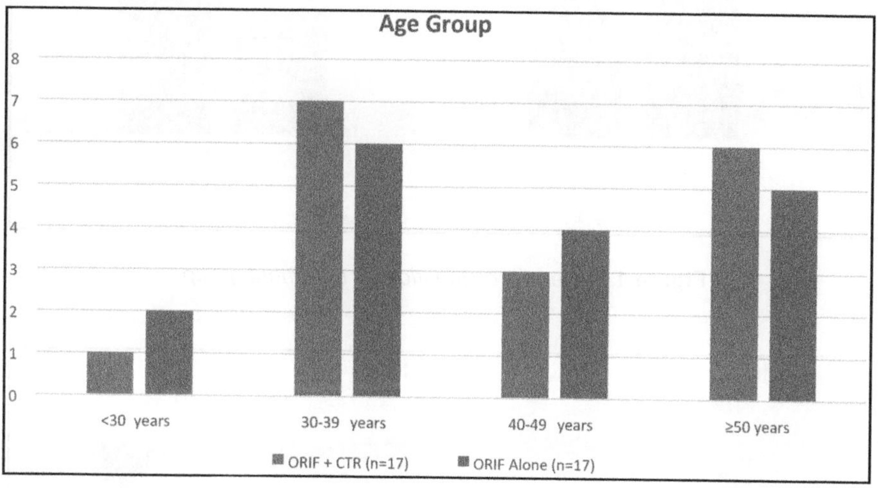

Figure 1.1. *Age categories comparison*

The age distribution of the groups was similar, and no notable differences were found (P = 0.715 in patients younger than 30), as shown in Figure 1.1. The highest number per cohort was the age group of 30–39 (41.2% versus 35.3%). Adolescents below 30 years made the least (5.9 versus 11.8). This shows that there is no selection bias on the basis of age.

There was no difference in gender distribution based on groups, with 70.6% of the ORIF + CTR, which consisted of men and 58.8% of ORIF-only, which consisted of men, as shown in Figure 1.2. The release group and ORIF-only group were 29.4 and 41.2%, respectively (women). The gender difference was not significant since the P-value was 0.715 and, hence, the demographics were equal.

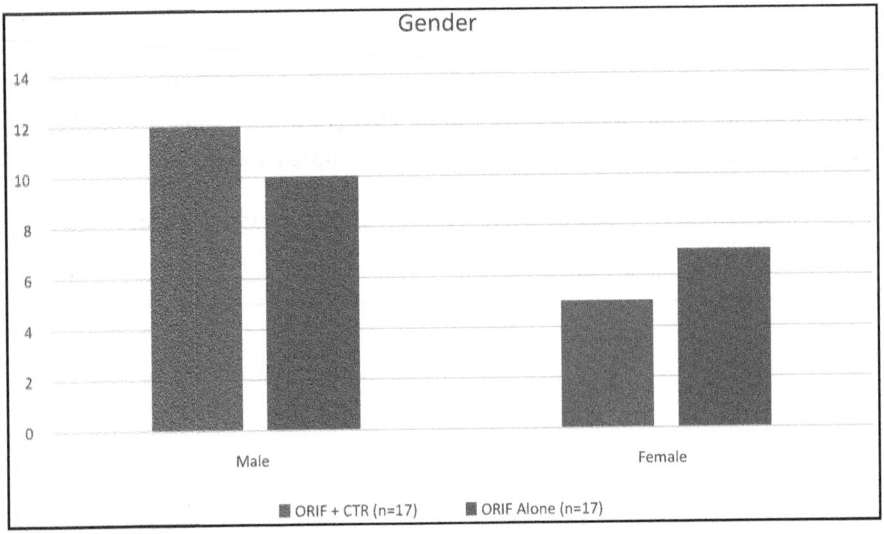

Figure 1.2. *Gender distribution by treatment group*

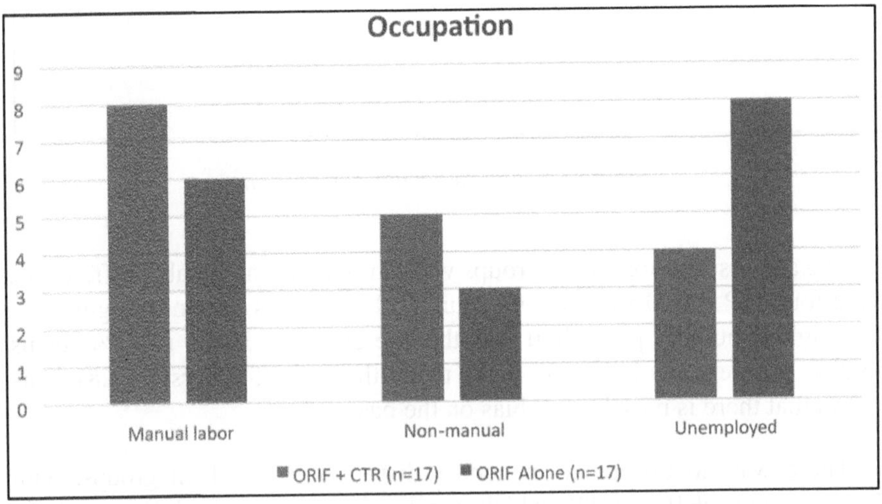

Figure 1.3. *Occupation distribution by treatment group*

The largest group of occupational activities in both arms was manual laborers (47.1% in ORIF + CTR versus 35.3% in ORIF-only) as shown in Figure 1.3. The unemployment rate among the patients of the ORIF-only group was higher (47.1 versus 23.5). The difference, even though not significant (P = 0.283), can have an impact on functional outcomes, as job demands also have effects on recovery and rehabilitation. Otherwise, there was no difference between groups on non-manual workers (29.4 versus 17.6).

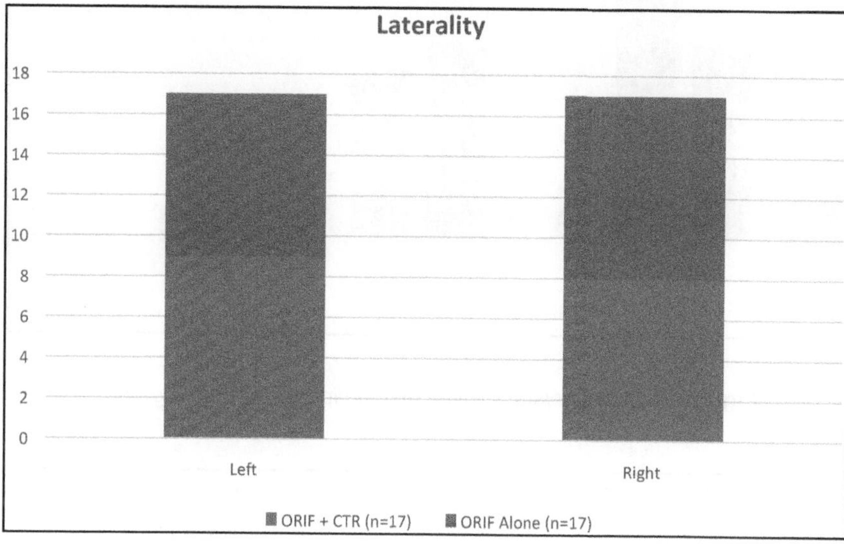

Figure 1.4. *Laterality distribution by treatment group*

Group-to-group laterality of injuries was almost the same. Left-sided injuries in the ORIF + CTR group were 52.9% and right-sided injuries were 52.9% in the ORIF-only group, as shown in Figure 1.4. No significant bias is ensured by the fact that the value of P equals 0.999. In the distribution of dominant versus non-dominant involvement of the hands, there is also an additional support for similar functional outcome measurements.

The mechanisms of injury were intergroup comparable. There was 41.2% and 52.9% variability in falls that happened in ORIF + CTR and ORIF-only cases, respectively. The percentage of ORIF + CTR injuries and ORIF-only injuries was 41.2 and 35.3, respectively, in road-traffic accidents. Assault represented one case only (neighborhood survey) in the mixed group. The

P-value of 0.621 does not reveal a significant difference, therefore indicating the same level of injuries during the baseline and eliminating confounding factors when comparing the results of treatment. The equal distribution increases the validity of postoperative comparisons.

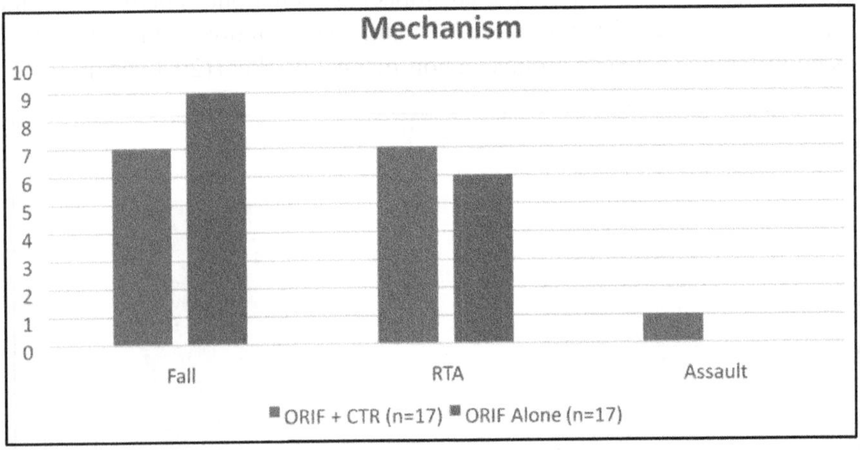

Figure 1.5. *Mechanism of injury distribution by treatment group*

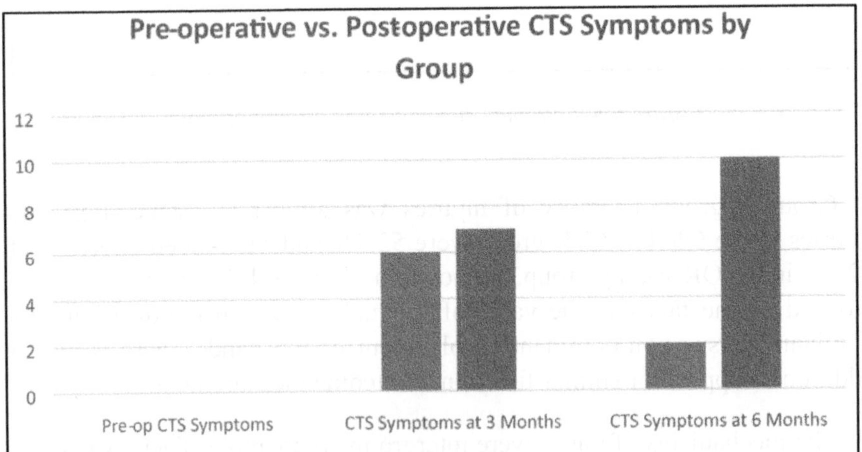

Figure 1.6. *Pre-operative versus postoperative CTS symptoms by group*

The patients did not have any preoperative CTS. Compared to the ORIF-only group, which was 58.8, the ORIF + CTR group had a significantly lower persistent CTS symptoms rate (58.8%, *p* = 0.008). The three-month results showed no difference (P = 0.500), but the addition of CTR was found to cushion the long-term CTS, as by six months, a significant difference had been observed.

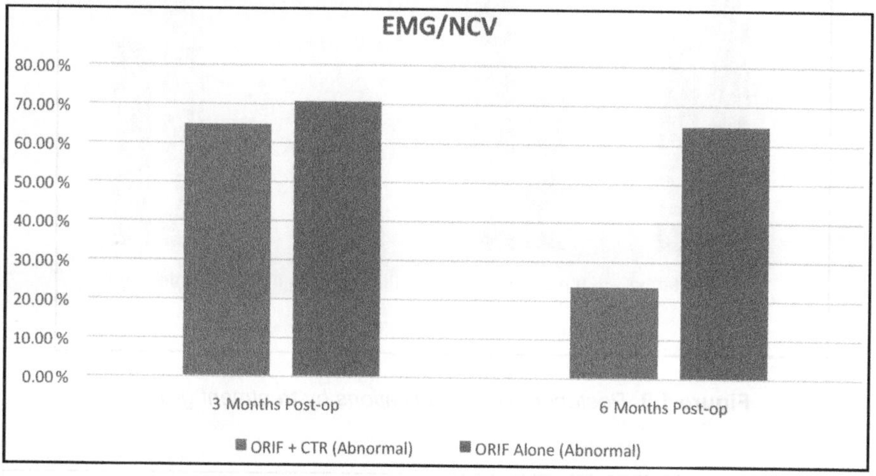

Figure 1.7. *Postoperative nerve conduction (EMG/NCV) abnormalities by treatment group*

At three months postoperation, abnormal findings were observed in 64.7% of ORIF + CTR patients compared to 70.6% of ORIF-alone patients. By six months, the ORIF + CTR group showed substantial improvement with only 23.5% abnormal cases, while the ORIF-alone group maintained a high rate of abnormal findings at 64.7%. This suggests that combined ORIF with CTR may lead to better long-term outcomes compared to ORIF alone, with a notable reduction in persistent abnormalities at the six-month follow-up.

There was no significant difference in the number of postoperative complications in the two cohorts (P > 0.05 in all of the comparisons). Nerve agitation was the case in 29.4% of ORIF + CTR and 23.5% of CTR cases (P = 0.500). The tendency toward tendon irritation was less in the mixed group (17.6% versus 29.4%; P = 0.480). Other major complications, plate loosening (5.9% versus 11.8%) and infection (29.4% versus 23.5%), also did not have significant differences. Therefore, the prophylactic use of CTR in

ORIF shows no significant risks in complication, and both methods seem to be safe, but larger studies are necessary to prove the results.

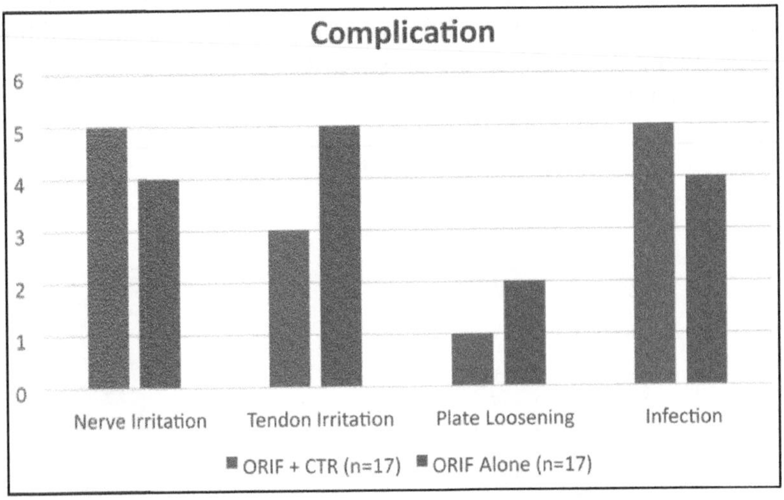

Figure 1.8. *Postoperative complications by treatment group*

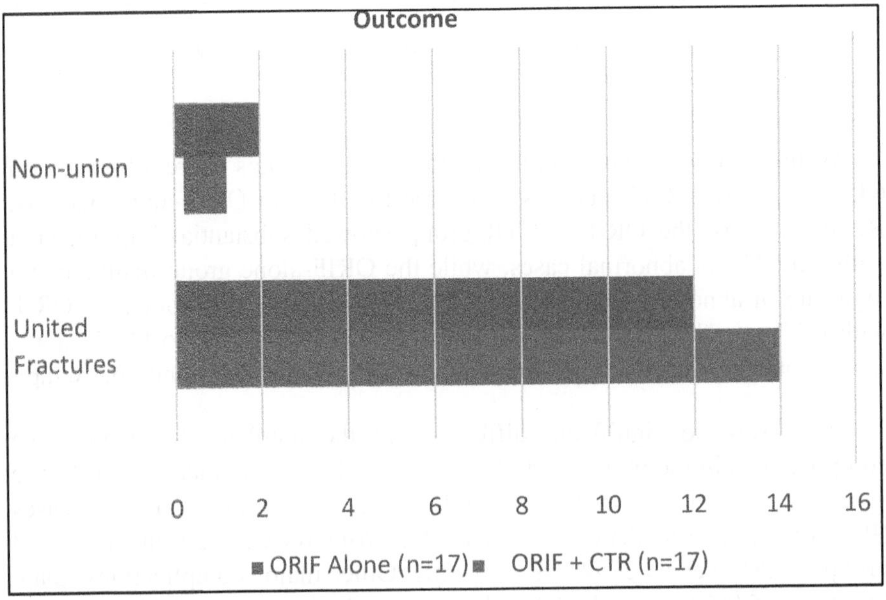

Figure 1.9. *Fracture union outcomes by treatment group*

The appositive rate of fracture union was 82.4% of the ORIF + CTR group and 70.6% of the ORIF-only group (P = 0.693). Rates of non-unions that combined the procedure were 5.9 a priori and 11.8 for ORIF. Even though the results indicate a potential usefulness of concurrent CTR, the reduced size of the sample does not allow the drawing of conclusions. In general, addition of CTR does not reduce fracture healing and may result in a small positive effect on union, which is to be evaluated in a larger study.

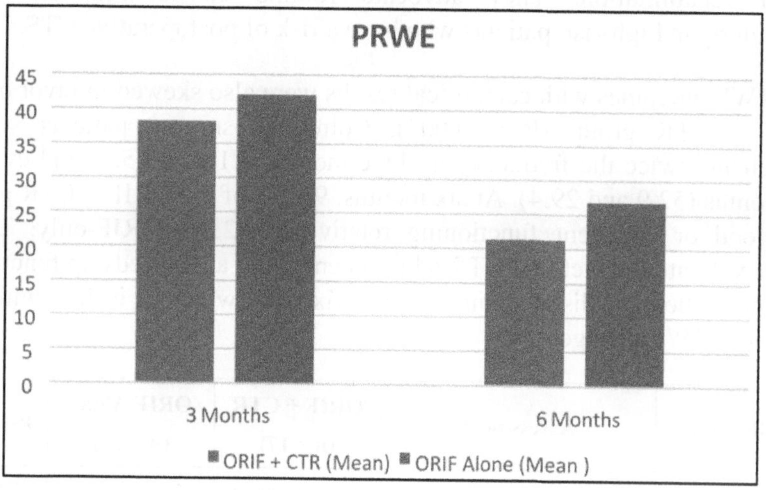

Figure 1.10. *PRWE scores by treatment group*

PRWE Category	Time Point	ORIF + CTR (n = 17)	ORIF Alone (n = 17)	P-value
Excellent (0–20)	3 Months	2 (11.8%)	1 (5.9%)	0.003
	6 Months	9 (52.9%)	5 (29.4%)	0.16
Good (21–40)	3 Months	10 (58.8%)	8 (47.1%)	0.73
	6 Months	7 (41.2%)	9 (52.9%)	0.73
Fair (41–60)	3 Months	5 (29.4%)	7 (41.2%)	0.71
	6 Months	1 (5.9%)	3 (17.6%)	0.60
Poor (> 60)	3 Months	0 (0%)	1 (5.9%)	1.00
	6 Months	0 (0%)	0 (0%)	Not applicable

Table 1.1. *PRWE outcomes by treatment group*

At both follow-ups, functional outcomes were greatly superior in the ORIF + CTR group. PRWE scores of the combined group (38.2 + 5.1) were worse (better) than those of the ORIF-only (42.1 + 6.3) three months postoperative (P = 0.042). The advantage increased at six months: the scores were 21.3 +/- 4.7 , 26.8 +/- 5.9 (P = 0.018). These findings suggest that prophylactic CTR in fracture fixation has real functional advantages, probably through maintenance of median nerve integrity and provision of an earlier rehabilitation. They advocate routine consideration of CTR particularly in high-risk patients who have a risk of postoperative CTS.

PRWE outcomes with categorical results were also skewed in favor of the ORIF + CTR group (P = 0.003). Combined surgery patients scored "Excellent" twice the frequency at three months (11.8 and 5.9) and even at six months (52.9 and 29.4). At six months, 94.1% of the ORIF + CTR group had good or excellent functioning relative to 82.3% ORIF-only. These results validate the fact that CTR addition enhances and speeds up functional recovery following distal radius fracture fixation, which is in line with the ongoing PRWE changes.

Follow-up	**Assessment**	**ORIF + CTR (n = 17)**	**ORIF Alone (n = 17)**	**P-value**
Two weeks	Wound healing	17/17 (100%)	17/17 (100%)	1.000
	Finger mobilization	17/17 (100%)	17/17 (100%)	1.000
Six weeks	Radiographic union	8/17 (47.1%)	6/17 (35.3%)	0.500
	Volar slab discontinued	17/17 (100%)	17/17 (100%)	1.000
	Pain score (VAS, mean)	3.2	4.1	0.032*
Three months	CTS symptoms persistent	3/17 (17.6%)	8/17 (47.1%)	0.041*
	EMG/NCV abnormal	4/17 (23.5%)	12/17 (70.6%)	0.003*
Six months	Fracture union achieved	14/17 (82.4%)	12/17 (70.6%)	0.693
	CTS symptoms persistent	2/17 (11.8%)	6/17 (35.3%)	0.046*

Table 1.2. *Postoperative recovery outcomes by treatment group*

Better results were also attained in the ORIF + CTR group in terms of multiple recovery measures. The pain scores were less at six weeks (VAS 3.2 versus 4.1; P = 0.032). The CTS symptoms were significantly diminished at three months (17.6% versus 47.1%; P = 0.041) and six months (11.8% versus 35.3%; P = 0.046). The nerve conduction abnormalities were reduced from 70.6% to 23.5% (P = 0.003). There were also similar wound healing and immobilization, but overall, there were higher final radionuclide union rates (82.4/70.6) and an earlier radionuclide union tendency (47.1/35.3) that was no longer significant (P > 0.05). All in all, CTR addition to ORIF does not worsen the fracture healing and enhances pain and neurologic outcomes.

Follow-up	Complication	ORIF + CTR (n = 17)	ORIF alone (n = 17)	*P*value
Two weeks	Infection	2 (11.8%)	1 (5.9%)	0.500
	Wound dehiscence	1 (5.9%)	2 (11.8%)	0.500
Six weeks	Tendon irritation	2 (11.8%)	4 (23.5%)	0.400
	Plate loosening	1 (5.9%)	3 (17.6%)	0.300
Three months	Nerve dysfunction	5 (29.4%)	4 (23.5%)	0.500
	Non-union	1 (5.9%)	3 (17.6%)	0.300
Six months	Chronic CTS symptoms	2/17 (11.8%)	6/17 (35.3%)	0.046*

Table 1.3. *Postoperative complications by treatment group*

The levels of complication in the ORIF + CTR group were always lower, but most of the differences were not found to be significant. Particularly, the ORIF alone group had achieved higher rates of plate loosening (17.6% versus 5.9%, *p* = 0.300), non-union (17.6% versus 5.9%, *p* = 0.300) and reoperations (11.8% versus 0%, *p* = 0.150). Early wound complications were equivalent in both groups, but the ORIF + CTR group had fewer tendon irritations (11.8% versus 23.5%) and persistent CTS symptoms (29.4% versus 41.2%). Attractive lack of reoperations in the combined procedure group implies that prophylactic CTR could decrease the necessity of the secondary interventions; however, the observations require additional studies of greater sizes.

Follow-up	Intervention	ORIF + CTR (n = 17)	ORIF Alone (n = 17)	*P*value
Two weeks	Sutures removed	17/17 (100%)	17/17 (100%)	1.000
	Passive ROM exercises	Initiated	Initiated	-
Six weeks	Active ROM exercises	17/17 (100%)	17/17 (100%)	1.000
	Strengthening exercises	10/17 (58.8%)	8/17 (47.1%)	0.500
Three months	Return to light work	12/17 (70.6%)	9/17 (52.9%)	0.300
Six months	Return tomanual labor	14/17 (82.4%)	11/17 (64.7%)	0.250

Table 1.4. *Rehabilitation progress and functional recovery by treatment group*

The two groups had comparable early rehabilitation interventions, where all patients achieved passive ROM after two weeks and active ROM after six weeks of rehabilitation (*P* = 1.000). The ORIF + CTR group also exhibited greater functional recovery, more frequent strengthening exercise at six weeks (58.8% versus 47.1%), earlier light employment at three months (70.6% versus 52.9%) and better employment at manual labor at six months (82.4% versus 64.7%). Although these differences were not statistically significant (i.e. *p* > 0.05), the general trend is similar, which indicates that combined CTR could have helped in the progress of the rehabilitation process, possibly because of decreased postoperative nerve symptoms. This is consistent with the previous advantage in functional recovery of the ORIF + CTR group, as they have high PRWE and lower complications in prior studies.

1.4. Discussion

The authors compared the results of two methods of surgery for fractures of the distal radius with the possible median nerve injury: one is associated with an ORIF with prophylactic CTR and the other one is associated with ORIF-only (Rothman et al. 2023). The evidence shows that the combination procedure (ORIF + CTR) is associated with a number of benefits, such as fewer nerve complications after surgery, higher rates of functional recovery and better pain control; moreover, there is no added risk of the procedure. These findings end up proving the possible advantage of the prevention of median nerve compression during the fracture fixation of the relevant patients.

Concerning the symptoms of CTS, the incidence of persistent CTS was significantly lower in patients undergoing ORIF with CTR (17.6% versus 47.1% at three months and 11.8% versus 58.3% at six months, respectively) than in patients undergoing ORIF alone. These results were further supported using electrophysiological measures, where an abnormal nerve conduction (EMG/NCV) was found in only 23.5% of the patients in the ORIF + CTR group as compared to 70.6% in the ORIF-only group (P = 0.003). These findings coincide with other reports by Lozano-Calderón et al. (2008), who revealed the increased rate of CTS after distal radius fractures and the better results offered by early or prophylactic CTR. Taken together, these results support the assumption that prophylactic CTR leads to lesser secondary median nerve compression due to post-traumatic edema, hemorrhaging or fracture-related displacement, and, therefore, better neurologic recovery and functional outcomes (Kashyap et al. 2024).

With regards to functional recovery and rehabilitation regarding postoperative pain scores, patients receiving ORIF with CTR showed reduced pain levels at six weeks (VAS 3.2 versus 4.1, P = 0.032); they were also able to initiate strengthening exercises sooner (58.8% versus 47.1%), and their return-to-work rates (especially in manual work) were higher at six weeks (82.4% versus 64.7%). The results are consistent with those of Grewal and MacDermid (2007), who found a delay in rehabilitation and worse functional outcomes in patients with persistent nerve symptoms. The lack of persistent median nerve compression in the ORIF + CTR group probably helped the patients with rehabilitation and led to better PRWE scores: 94.1% reported a good or excellent result versus 82.3% in the ORIF-alone group (Deng et al. 2021).

Even though not all of the differences were statistically significant, the ORIF + CTR measured lower rates of complications and reoperations, a reduced number of plate loosening (5.90 versus 17.60), non-union rates (5.90 versus 17.60) and zero cases of reoperations as opposed to 11.80 cases of reoperation wherein the ORIF-alone group had a higher rate of reoperations. Such tendencies are justified by the earlier surveys showing that untreated CTS may be a reason to conduct a secondary surgery and augment the postoperative morbidity. Some of the studies have raised doubts in regard to using prophylactic CTR regularly, but most of them were based on low-risk fracture shapes (Kumar et al. 2026). Conversely, the current findings highlight the significance of the risk-stratified method, especially in patients who have intense fracture displacement or comminution.

1.5. Conclusion

Volar plate fixation is the most popular method of fixing distal end radius fractures to reinstate the wrist anatomy and functionality, but the median nerve complications that follow surgery, especially CTS, are another major issue of concern. This chapter evidenced that patients that have undergone ORIF with CTR have better neurological and functional outcomes than those who are only receiving ORIF. The overall process showed a better result in the incidence of persistent CTS symptoms and better nerve conduction results at the follow-up, as it shows an effective protection and recovery of the median nerve functioning. Functionally, the patients who have experienced ORIF together with CTR have higher PRWE scores, decreased postoperative pain and a faster recovery to daily and occupational activities. Notably, the risk of getting surgical complications was not elevated by the introduction of CTR, which proves that this method is safe and does not negatively influence the Achilles tendon union of fractures. The comparative analysis, assisted with AI, enhanced the outcome assessment, as the results incorporated the clinical, electrophysiological and functional results. In summary, selective prophylactic CTR in volar plating is a safe and effective method that can help patients who are vulnerable to developing postoperative CTS, and it should be recommended to be included in personal surgical strategies in distal radius fractures.

1.6. References

Barnes, J.I., Paci, G., Zhuang, T., Baker, L.C., Asch, S.M., Kamal, R.N. (2021). Cost-effectiveness of open versus endoscopic carpal tunnel release. *JBJS*, 103(4), 343–355.

Buijze, G.A., Jupiter, J., Chammas, M. (eds) (2021). *Distal Radius Fractures: Evidence-Based Management*. Elsevier, Amsterdam.

Coon, M., Denisiuk, M., Woodbury, D., Best, B., Vaidya, R. (2022). Closed fracture treatment in adults, when is it still relevant? *Spartan Medical Research Journal*, 7(1), 28060.

Deng, Z., Wu, J., Tang, K., Shu, H., Wang, T., Li, F., Nie, M. (2021). In adults, early mobilization may be beneficial for distal radius fractures treated with open reduction and internal fixation: A systematic review and meta-analysis. *Journal of Orthopaedic Surgery and Research*, 16(1), 691.

Grewal, R. and MacDermid, J.C. (2007). The risk of adverse outcomes in extra-articular distal radius fractures is increased with malalignment in patients of all ages but mitigated in older patients. *J. Hand Surg. Am.*, 32(7), 962–970.

Hall, M.J., Ostergaard, P.J., Rozental, T.D. (2021). Outcome measurement for distal radius fractures. *Hand Clinics*, 37(2), 215–227.

Hassan, N.A., Elsawy, N.A., Kotb, H.H., El-Hamid, M.M., El Emairy, W.S., Kholosy, H.M. (2021). Evaluation of outcome after primary median and/or ulnar nerve(s) repair at wrist: Clinical, functional, electrophysiologic, and ultrasound study. *Egyptian Rheumatology and Rehabilitation*, 48(1), 48.

John, A., Rossettie, S., Rafael, J., Cox, C., Ducic, I., Mackay, B. (2022). Assessment of motor function in peripheral nerve injury and recovery. *Orthopedic Reviews*, 14(3), 37578.

Kashyap, S., Ambade, R., Landge, S., Salwan, A. (2024). Impact of surgical timing on fracture healing in tibial shaft injuries: A comparative review of intramedullary nailing techniques. *Cureus*, 16(10), 1–14.

Kew, M.E. and Brockmeier, S.F. (2021). Complications following proximal biceps tenodesis. In *The Management of Biceps Pathology: A Clinical Guide from the Shoulder to the Elbow*, Romeo, A.A., Erickson, B.J., Griffin, J.W. (eds). Springer, Cham, 225–234.

Kumar, A., Batta, P., Rathore, P.S., Ahuja, S. (2025). Secure healthcare data sharing and attack detection framework using radial basis neural network. *Scientific Reports*, 15(1), 15432.

Kumar, A., Batta, P., Ahuja, S., Rathore, P.S. (eds) (2026). *AI-Driven Innovations in Physiotherapy and Oncology 2*. ISTE Ltd, London and Wiley, Hoboken, NJ.

Lacinski, R.A., Steller, J.G., Anderson, A., Nelson, A.M. (2024). Harnessing artificial intelligence for medical diagnosis and treatment during space exploration missions. Thesis, University of California, Irvine.

Laohaprasitiporn, P., Boonchai, K., Monteerarat, Y., Limthongthang, R., Vathana, T. (2022). Comparative clinical and radiographic outcomes between early and delayed wrist mobilization after volar fixed-angle plate fixation of distal radius fracture. *Scientific Reports*, 12(1), 9648.

Lozano-Calderón, S.A., Souer, S., Mudgal, C., Jupiter, J.B., Ring, D. (2008). Wrist mobilization following volar plate fixation of fractures of the distal part of the radius. *J. Bone Joint Surg. Am.*, 90(6), 1297–1304.

Maccagnano, G., Noia, G., Vicenti, G., Baglioni, M., Masciale, M.R., Cassano, G.D., Vitiello, R., Moretti, B., Pesce, V. (2021). Volar locking plate versus external fixation in distal radius fractures: A meta-analysis. *Orthopedic Reviews*, 13(1), 9147.

Malakootian, M., Soveizi, M., Gholipour, A., Oveisee, M. (2023). Pathophysiology, diagnosis, treatment, and genetics of carpal tunnel syndrome: A review. *Cellular and Molecular Neurobiology*, 43(5), 1817–1831.

Mehta, S.P., Karagiannopoulos, C., Pepin, M.E., Ballantyne, B.T., Michlovitz, S., MacDermid, J.C., Grewal, R., Martin, R.L. (2024). Distal radius fracture rehabilitation: Clinical practice guidelines linked to the international classification of functioning, disability, and health from the academy of orthopaedic physical therapy and academy of hand and upper extremity physical therapy of the American physical therapy association. *Journal of Orthopaedic & Sports Physical Therapy*, 54(9), CPG1-78.

Ochen, Y., Peek, J., van der Velde, D., Beeres, F.J., van Heijl, M., Groenwold, R.H., Houwert, R.M., Heng, M. (2020). Operative vs nonoperative treatment of distal radius fractures in adults: A systematic review and meta-analysis. *JAMA Network Open*, 3(4), e203497.

Pergolizzi, J.V. Jr., Le Quang, J.A., Magnusson, P., Varrassi, G. (2023). Identifying risk factors for chronic postsurgical pain and preventive measures: A comprehensive update. *Expert Review of Neurotherapeutics*, 23(12), 1297–1310.

Reimann, J. and Wijesekera, L. (2022). Diagnostic tests in the acute setting: Strengths and limitations. In *Emergencies in Neuromuscular Disorders*, Damian, M. and de Visser, M. (eds). Springer, Cham, 19–77.

Rothman, A., Samineni, A.V., Sing, D.C., Zhang, J.Y., Stein, A.B. (2023). Carpal tunnel release performed during distal radius fracture surgery. *Journal of Wrist Surgery*, 12(03), 211–217.

Williams, K.S. (2024). Evaluations of artificial intelligence and machine learning algorithms in neurodiagnostics. *Journal of Neurophysiology*, 131(5), 825–831.

2

Trigger Digits: Steroid Injection Versus Percutaneous Release Using AI-Based Outcome Analysis

Trigger digit or stenosing tenosynovitis is a very common hand disorder that is brought about by mechanical obstruction of the flexor tendon at the A1 pulley. Functional impairment, blockage and locking are some of the results of this blockage. Local steroid injections by doctors or percutaneous release of the A1 pulley is typically the treatment for it, although the comparative efficacy of these procedures is a controversial subject. Artificial intelligence (AI) was used in this chapter in order to compare the two techniques. We conducted a prospective cohort study of adults and undertook a routine clinical assessment, a Disabilities of the Arm, Shoulder and Hand (DASH) scale and the Visual Analogue Scale (VAS) enhancement of the pain at set follow-up periods. The patterns of symptom resolution, recurrence, function and complications are defined by the AI-assisted data analysis. The findings indicated that both techniques provided pain relief in the initial stages; however, the percutaneous release provided excellent relief with respect to pain, functional outcome, recurrence and longevousness. There was excellent safety of treatments and no neurovascular or infectious complications. These results indicate that outcome analysis with the assistance of AI can be realized to generate better comparisons and that percutaneous release can be the efficacious and long-term alternative among moderate-to-severe disease patients or those with recurrence following conservative treatment.

2.1. Introduction

Stenosing tenosynovitis is one of the most common hand conditions, which is encountered commonly in surgical and orthopedic practice, also

---

Chapter written by Anshuraj JAGDALE and Jineshwar S. KAPALE.

For a color version of all the figures in this chapter, see www.iste.co.uk/kumar/orthopedic1.zip.

referred to as trigger digit (Ng et al. 2023). It is characterized by pain, tenderness, clicking, locking or fixed flexion of the affected finger due to a disruption of the sliding of the flexor tendon through a reduced A1 pulley. It is found in approximately 2–3% of the general population and in as high as 10% of diabetic individuals, and it occurs more often in the middle-aged and elderly women (Ciarambino et al. 2022). The ensuing functional impairment may grossly interfere with everyday life and also work, which stresses the importance of promptly and efficiently treating impairment.

A failure between the size of the flexor tendon and fibro-osseous tunnel formed by the A1 pulley is the fundamental pathology of trigger digit (Schmitt et al. 2022). Referred to as hypertrophy and fibrocartilaginous metaplasia, repeated mechanical stress, friction and microtrauma result in the pulley hypertrophying. The result is mechanical blockage in tending to the movements of the tendons. Histopathology reveals pulley thickening, degeneration, unorganized collagen, chondroid metaplasia and inflammatory cell invasion (Kissin 2024), all of which interrupt smooth tendon gliding, and an effect of which is the classic symptoms of triggering and locking.

In the case of patients, they tend to manifest clinical features of pain in the base of the digit, morning stiffness, tenderness in the area of the metacarpophalangeal joint and a nodule on the hand (Kumar et al. 2026). The further evolution of the condition enhances the triggering, and in severe cases, a fixed flexion contracture occurs. The systems of Green and Quinnell are known to grade severity and thus the action to be taken and the prevalent way of assessing the outcomes.

Trigger digit management has both conservative and surgical management. Some of the conservative practices include activity modification, non-steroidal anti-inflammatory medication, splint and injecting local corticosteroid into the sheath around the flexor tendon (Pathak et al. 2022).

In most patients, the first-line treatment is steroid injection, which is not complicated, cheap and less invasive. It decreases the tendon sheath and pulley inflammation, which enhances tendon glide. There is a success rate of 60–90%, but recurrence is more common, especially with diabetic patients, who experience long-term symptoms or have higher disease grades.

Retained symptomatology, recurrence of symptoms after injection and severe triggering of symptoms are the conditions when surgical management is prescribed. Surgical interventions are open A1 pulley release and percutaneous release (PR). Open release has the benefit of direct visualization and good decompression; however, it may cause scar tenderness, infection and delayed recovery, as well as increase the cost. Percutaneous A1 pulley release has become a relatively uninvolved substitute, which can be conducted using local anesthesia as an outpatient procedure. This method is fast in giving the symptom a solution, early rehabilitation and reduced morbidity with precise anatomy understanding, as the A1 pulley is split using salient features on the surface.

Although there is a lot of literature that would prove the efficacy of both steroid injection and PR, both methods are still subject to controversy regarding highly effective treatment. Steroid injections are not as invasive but recur more often and are ineffective with diabetic patients. PR is more conclusive but creates problems of insufficient release as well as neurovascular damage, particularly to the border digits. The majority of comparative research works are based on traditional statistics, which might not be able to explain the intricate trends of symptom development, reoccurrence and functional restoration.

Introducing artificial intelligence (AI) into the work of clinics brings opportunities to new outcomes analysis. The AI-based approaches automatically test multidimensional clinical data, detect latent patterns and enhance the quality of comparisons of treatment modalities.

The use of AI in orthopedic and hand surgery has demonstrated potential in terms of outcome prediction, risk stratification and decision support, but little information exists on the application of this tool in trigger digit management (Lalehzarian et al. 2021).

The proposed study is an attempt to compare local steroid injection (LSI) and percutaneous A1 pulley release of trigger digits with AI-based outcome measurement. Through integrating clinical, functional and pain examination parameters, we will test the effectiveness of the treatment methods, re-occurrence, sustained symptom improvement and complication. The application of AI analysis should result in an increased level of objectivity and an overall stronger comparison between modalities (Changhez et al. 2024).

Knowledge of the comparative advantages and drawbacks of these interventions is vital toward maximum patient outcomes and evidence-based clinical decision-making. This study can provide a holistic evaluation of the effectiveness of treatments in the control of trigger digits by combining prospective clinical evaluation with an analysis provided by ANI.

The study compares LSI and percutaneous A1 pulley release with each other to compare and contrast their effectiveness in reduction of symptoms and hand functionality. It also investigates recurrence rates after treatment, symptom relief durability and longevity, and fullness of tendon release that has occurred with the percutaneous method as either partial or full release. The rates of treatment-associated complications that include tendon or neurovascular bundle injury and postoperative infection are also assessed. This study seeks to offer evidence-based information on the best and safest treatment option for trigger digits by systematically and objectively assessing these inflammations by clinical and functional means.

2.2. Literature review

Stenosing tenosynovitis or trigger digit is a common hand complaint leading to a stiff finger that freezes into position or catches or even clicks as the patient bends or straightens the finger. The problem will occur in cases where the flexor tendon is excessively wide with reference to the A1 pulley around the metacarpophalangeal joint (Ng et al. 2023). It is prevalent most often in middle-aged and older adults, particularly women and individuals with diabetes or rheumatoid arthritis. The pathophysiology of the disease typically includes thickening of the tendon sheath and A1 pulley, and they inhibit the movement of the tendon and impair the functions of the hands.

Over the years, different treatments, such as basic conservative and surgery-related ones, have been proposed, their primary goal being to alleviate pain, restore movement and prevent its recurrence.

2.3. Conservative management: LSI

The procedure of injecting a steroid into the tendon sheath is one of the most commonly used as a first-line intervention due to being a minimally invasive procedure, which can be performed effortlessly, at minimal cost, and, in many cases, will result in a significant amount of relief. The steroids decrease the inflammation, decrease the swollen sheath and help the tendon to slide much more easily. Research and a critical review indicate that 70–80% of cases are responsive, particularly when the trigger is early and is not accompanied by severe locking or fixed deformity (Zorzi 2024). Nonetheless, symptoms reoccur within months in a number of patients. Recurrence may occur up to 50% in six months, especially with insoluble steroids such as triamcinolone, with soluble steroids such as dexamethasone or betamethasone showing a lower recurrence with increased likelihood of reduced overall efficacy.

Several factors determine the success of steroid injections: specific steroid type and dosage, accuracy of the injection method, severity of trigger, length of symptoms and other health conditions of a patient (Hollins et al. 2022). An analysis of almost 900 patients served as a retrospective analysis to show that there are inconsistent success rates and that it relied on the steroid of our choice; dexamethasone reproduced higher recurrence as compared to certain other agents. Whereas, the process of injections is straightforward and relatively harmless, re-injury may weaken or atrophically affect the tendon, and the effectiveness of steroid injections tends to depreciate over time; this is the reason why it is difficult to predict what long-term solution can be found (Freedman et al. 2022).

2.4. PR: technique and outcomes

The A1 pulley was initially originally described as performed by Lothario in 1958 through PR. The operation is non-surgical in nature and is conducted by local anesthetic use of a needle or fine blade (Sayed et al. 2024). The mechanical block to tendon movement is removed head-on by the cut of the constricting pulley technique. The surgery is possible as an outpatient, the process itself lasting just a couple of minutes, and early mobilization is possible. Due to the fact that it is carried out without direct visualization, it is necessary to have detailed anatomical knowledge and a careful technique to prevent the damage of nerve or blood vessels.

Evidence from comparative studies generally supports the high efficacy of PR. A prospective randomized trial comparing percutaneous A1 pulley release with steroid injection demonstrated that PR was associated with significantly lower recurrence rates than steroid treatment at six-month follow-up (0% recurrence in percutaneous group versus ~ 11% in steroid group). Patients undergoing PR also had less pain on motion at six months, although the steroid group showed faster improvement in range of motion and grip strength at one month. In addition, randomized clinical trials (e.g. in adult patients in Nepal) have shown that PR is superior in functional improvement and pain reduction compared to steroid injection, with statistically significant differences in outcomes such as Quinnell's classification and VAS pain scores (Karki et al. 2025).

2.5. Comparative efficacy: steroid injection versus PR

Several studies directly comparing the two modalities support the notion that PR generally yields better medium-term outcomes than steroid injections in terms of lower recurrence, greater long-term functional improvement and better patient satisfaction. Analysis of extensive series of patients indicates that PR is more successful compared to the use of steroids only. PR has a pooled success of approximately 30–94% versus approximately 65% using steroid injection alone.

Injections of steroids are only temporary in the short run and less effective in the long-run, and most patients ultimately undergo surgery due to persistence or recurrence of the syphilitic symptoms (Stone et al. 2021).

Subsequent prospective comparisons indicate that although pain tends to change at a more rapid rate with a steroid injection, PR shows a lasting removal of clicking and locking. It also has minimal rates of late recurrence and reduced re-interventions (Levine et al. 2022). Observational and randomized studies indicate that patient satisfaction, visual analogy scale scores and functional outcomes are more likely to be greater using PR.

2.6. Complications and safety considerations

Both approaches may be problematic. In the case of steroid injections, weakening or rupture of tendons, which frequently occurs with ongoing injection use, color changes in the skin of the area of injections, local infection and possible temporary symptoms aggravation are the most frequent issues. To avoid these problems, clinicians tend to restrict repeat injections.

The PR is blind, and therefore, it has risks. These involve subcomplete release of the pulley, rupture of the digital nerves, tendon rupture and persevering triggering. However, there are very rare cases of serious complications in case the procedure is performed by skilled professionals, and it has minor and temporary problems in most cases. Percussion recurrence has also been described in recurrence; certain long-term studies indicate recurrence rates of up to approximately 5%. Percutaneous release requires precise technique and extensive postoperative immobilization (Chanthanapodi and Aodsup 2025).

2.7. Meta-analyses and systematic reviews

Surgical releases, be they percutaneous or open, are always favored in high-level evidence based on systematic reviews and meta-analyses to achieve long-term success over steroid injection use. Reviews indicate more success and satisfaction with surgical release and have no difference in the level of overall complication. A single meta-analysis that investigated PR with or without concomitant steroid injection discovered that the addition of a steroid would implement a minor reduction to the postoperative disability, yet the general satisfaction, recurrence and pain would be the same. Therefore, it is possible to note that both interventions could be safe and useful when chosen correctly (Levine et al. 2022).

2.8. Clinical implications and future directions

Overall, the literature justifies the use of LSI as a minimal invasive and early trigger digits treatment algorithm. This would particularly be appropriate in those patients who prefer conservative treatment or have contraindications to surgery (Patrinely et al. 2021). However, PR is generally preferred for Grade II–III trigger fingers, recurrent cases after steroid injection, or when long-term resolution is prioritized, given its favorable efficacy and functional outcomes.

Future research, ideally through larger multicenter randomized trials with standardized outcome measures and longer follow-up durations, is needed to refine risk stratification and optimize decision-making criteria regarding when to choose steroid injection versus PR in diverse patient populations.

2.9. Materials and methods

2.9.1. *Materials and method of selection*

Approval for this investigation was obtained from the authors' Institutional Review Board and informed consent from all patients in KIMSDU, Karad Hospital, India. A total of twenty patients were treated, and clinical and functional outcome assessments were performed. The sample was selected randomly, with randomization done using the chit method, from all of the patients who satisfied the inclusion and exclusion criteria, to minimize selection bias.

2.9.2. *Conduction of study*

Patients were enlisted in this study after taking a careful thorough history, clinical examination and laboratory investigations wherever necessary and a USG scan if required.

The patients eligible for the study were informed and briefed regarding the above study, and proper informed, valid, written consent was taken for participation in the study.

Patient follow-up was conducted on day 14, one month and two months post-treatment to check for tendon relief, improvement in flexion, injury to tendon/vessels, infection, recurrence, restriction and triggering.

– *Study design*: prospective study.

– *Study duration*: 18 months.

2.9.2.1. *Patient selection criteria*

The inclusion and exclusion criteria to select the patients for the study are as follows:

– Inclusion criteria:

1) Age twenty years and above.

2) Professional tenosynovitis.

3) Known case of rheumatoid arthritis who have triggering.

4) Diabetic patients with good glycemic control.

5) Patients in whom conservative treatment failed.

– Exclusion criteria:

1) Patients below the age of twenty years.

2) Uncontrolled diabetics/diabetics with poor glycemic control.

3) Localized infections.

2.9.3. *Sample size*

The formula used for determining the sample size is as follows:

N = (za+zb)2 (S12+S22) / (m2-m1)2

$Z_a = 1.96$ Type I error with 5% level of significance.

$Z_b = 1.64$ Type II error with 95% power.

$n = (1.96 + 1.64)^2 \times (0.6^2 \times 1.8^2) / (4.6\text{-}0.8)^2 = 3.23\ n \approx 3$

Taking at least 10 in both groups:

[n = 10 + 10 = 20]

2.9.4. *Statistical analysis*

Twenty patients with trigger fingers were recruited in the current study. IBM SPSS Statistics version 29.0 was used to analyze the data so that all of the variables have been dealt with in a robust manner. Frequency and percentages of categorical variables and means and standard deviations of continuous variables were used as descriptive statistics. Unpaired two-sample t-tests were used to compare two independent groups. The categories of data were examined using chi-square or Fisher's testing, as suitable. The P-value of less than 0.05 was used as a sign of statistical significance in all tests.

2.10. Observation and results

2.10.1. *Age distribution*

The sample size of 20 participants was between 38 and 70 years, with an average age of 52.9 years (SD = 11.86). The majority of the patients fell within the late 40s to mid-60s. The minimum age was 38 years, and the maximum age was 70 years. The median age of the population between 41.5 and 65.5 years made the majority fall within the middle-aged to elderly age group.

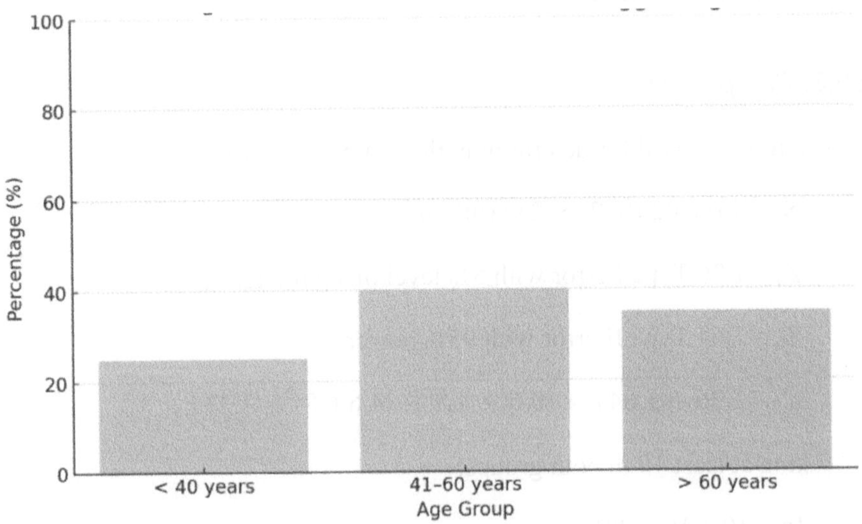

Figure 2.1. *Age distribution of patients with trigger digits*

The age groups 41–50 years and 61–70 years were the most represented, with the proportion of 25 and 35 cases as the age estimates, respectively. This distribution is consistent with the available literature that trigger finger occurs most frequently in the fifth and sixth decades of life, suggesting an increased clinical load among middle-aged adults.

2.10.2. *Sex distribution*

Of the 20 patients, 12 (60%) were females and 8 (40%) were males. The same distribution is reflected in the epidemiological pattern according to which finger is more common among females, in particular, the middle-age group.

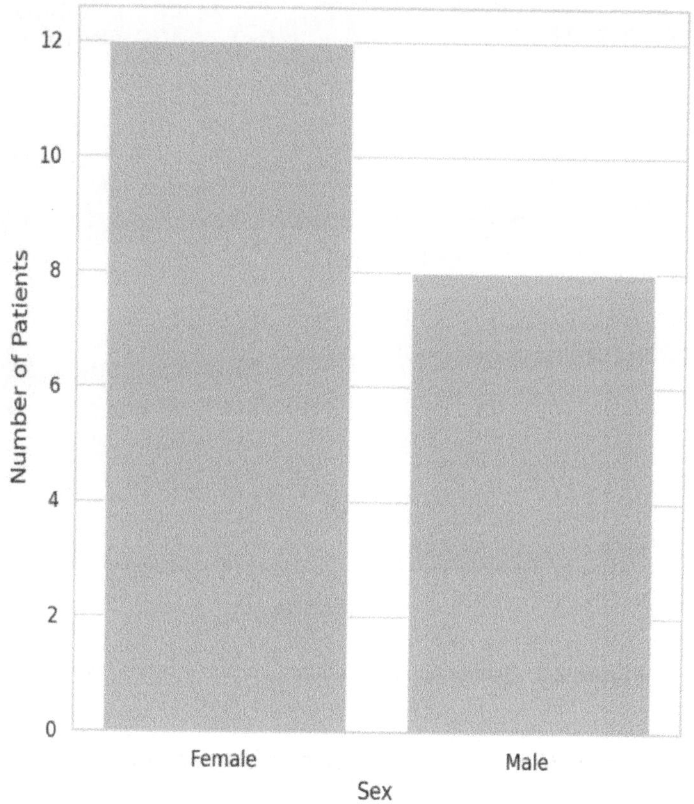

Figure 2.2. *Sex distribution of patients*

2.10.3. *Side distribution*

Dominance and involvement of hands

Among the study participants, 13 patients (65%) were left-hand dominant, while 7 patients (35%) were right-hand dominant. Regarding the affected hand, the right hand was involved in 11 cases (55%), whereas the left hand was involved in 9 cases (45%). Cross-tabulation of the dominant and affected hands indicated that both dominant and non-dominant hands were susceptible to involvement. This suggests that hand dominance alone may not determine the site of involvement. Other contributing factors, such as repetitive strain or local anatomical predisposition, may also influence the occurrence of the condition.

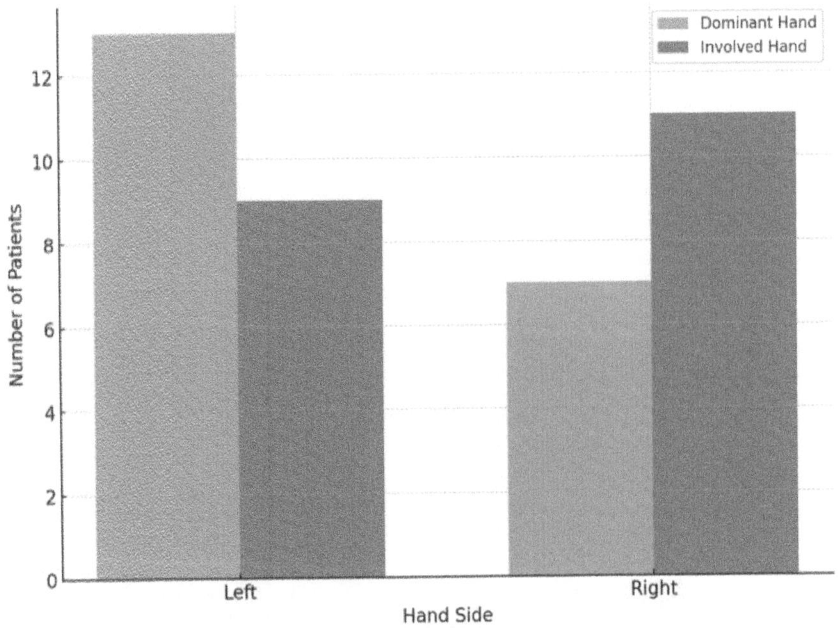

Figure 2.3. *Distribution of dominant versus involved hand*

2.10.4. *Pre-operative analysis of Green's grading*

Pre-operative assessment of Green's Grading revealed that the majority of patients presented with moderate to severe involvement. Of all of the

20 patients evaluated, 12 (60%) were found to be Grade III. Grade II accounted for 4 (20%) of the cases. An equal proportion, four patients (20%), presented with Grade IV, the most severe form, marked by fixed flexion contracture of the digit. None of the patients were Grade I.

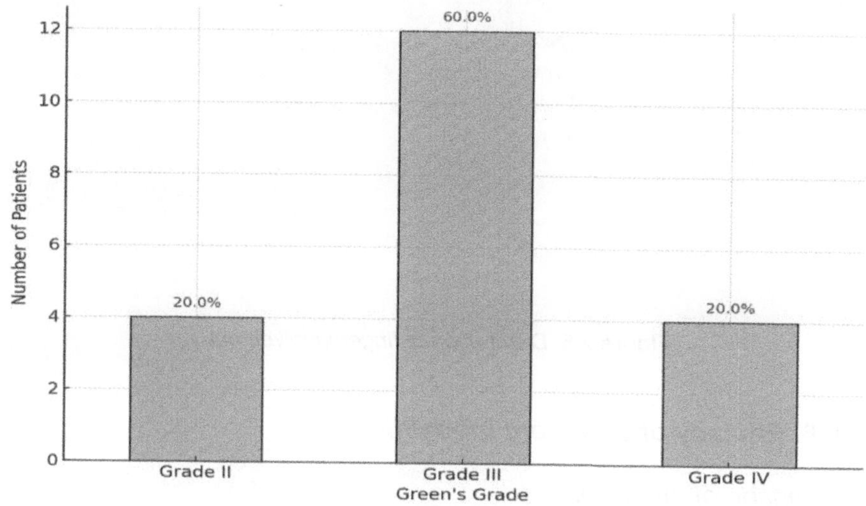

Figure 2.4. *Pre-operative analysis of Green's grading*

2.10.5. *Finger involvement*

In this study, a detailed analysis of finger involvement was carried out to determine the pattern of digit distribution in trigger finger cases. The most affected joint was the middle finger, which constituted 35% of all affected; the next was the ring finger (30%), index finger (20%) and finally the little finger (15%). None of the participants had an impact on the thumb. This is in line with the previous research findings that reveal greater vulnerability in the middle and ring fingers to recurrent mechanical stress during its involvement in grasping and power grip, contributing to the risk of stenosing tenosynovitis at the A1 pulley.

The fact that the findings have consistently been similar to previous studies would enable the idea that repetitive mechanical strain on some of the digits predisposes them to trigger finger.

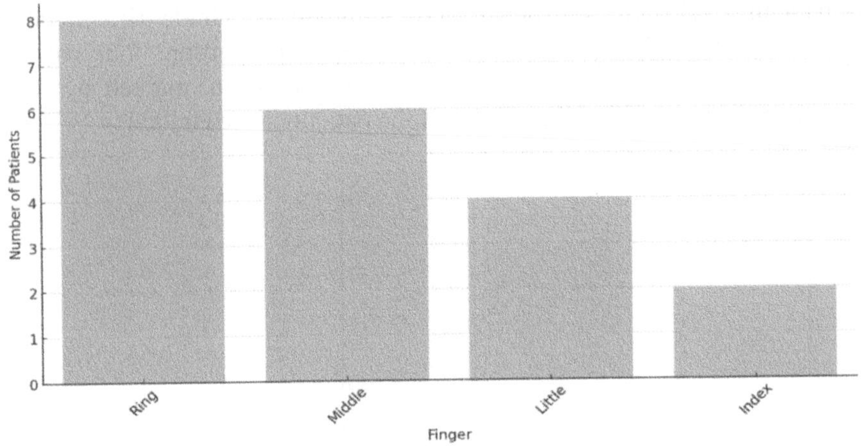

Figure 2.5. *Distribution of finger involvement*

2.10.6. *Efficacy of treatment modalities*

Comparison of effectiveness

The effectiveness of local steroid injection was compared with PR by evaluating the DASH (Disabilities of the Arm, Shoulder and Hand) and VAS (Visual Analogue Scale) scores. These scores were recorded before treatment and subsequently at two weeks, one month, and two months after the initiation of treatment to assess clinical improvement over time.

Both groups showed clinical improvement, but the percutaneous release group exhibited a more pronounced and sustained benefit. The mean DASH score in the percutaneous group decreased from 54.3 preoperatively to 30.6 at 2 months (43.7% reduction), while the steroid group showed a decline from 58.0 to 45.5 (21.6% reduction). Although differences at 2 weeks ($p = 0.73$) and 1 month ($p = 0.29$) were not statistically significant, the 2-month difference showed statistical significance ($p = 0.003$).

VAS pain scores followed a similar trend. In the percutaneous group, scores dropped from 7.0 preoperatively to 2.4 at two months, compared to a decline from 7.4 to only 5.8 in the steroid group. The differences between the two groups were statistically significant at one month ($P = 0.048$) and highly significant at two months ($P < 0.0001$), although not at two weeks ($P = 0.15$). These findings indicate that while both treatments offer early symptom relief, PR yields significantly superior long-term functional improvement and pain reduction, supporting its efficacy as the preferred treatment modality for trigger digits.

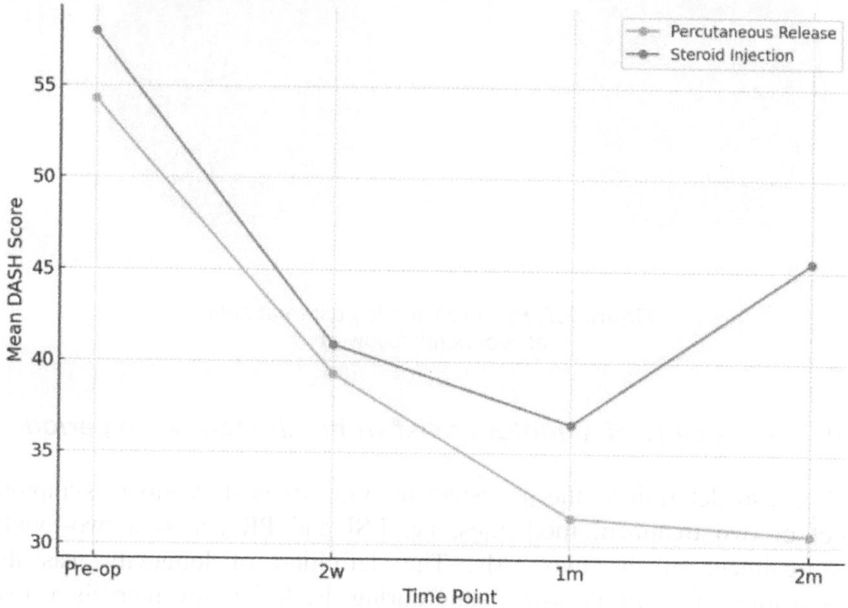

Figure 2.6. *An efficacy of treatment modalities (dash score)*

2.10.7. *Recurrence rate post-treatment*

A chi-square test was conducted to estimate the association between treatment modality and symptom recurrence at the two-month follow-up. Of all of the patients managed with PR, none (0/10) exhibited recurrence, whereas recurrence was seen in 50% (5/10) of all of the patients who got LSI. The chi-square test provided 0.0389 (df = 1) and 0.0389 (chi-square = 4.27), respectively, and this shows that there is post-hoc significance in the association between the modalities of treatment and recurrence rate.

Clinical evidence indicated that PR showed better results in prolonging symptomatic relief rates and reducing recurrence rates after two months, and this could be considered a more efficient and permanent alternative than LSI.

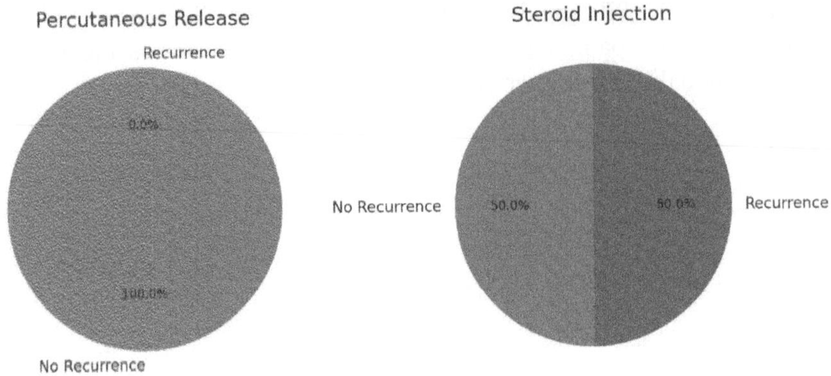

Figure 2.7. *Recurrence rate post-treatment at two-month follow-up*

2.10.8. *Longevity of symptom relief within the follow-up period*

We also determined the persistent duration of post-treatment symptom relief of two treatment modalities, i.e. LSI and PR across a two-month post-treatment of the two TMs. The definition of longevity was the preservation of a symptom-free state during the follow-up intervals at two weeks, one month and two-month follow-ups.

In the PR group, ten out of ten patients (100% reported no exudation of the same during the entire two-month follow-up) reported long-term relief. The LSI group, in contrast, was five of ten patients (50%) who returned to the symptoms within the same period.

To check for the correlation between treatment modality and sustained symptom relief, a chi-square test was performed and the analysis revealed a statistically significant difference between the two groups (χ^2 = 4.27, P = 0.0389), demonstrating that PR was significantly more effective in maintaining early symptom resolution.

These findings support the short-term superiority of PR in terms of symptom longevity, although this study does not allow conclusions to be drawn regarding the long-term durability beyond two months due to the limited follow-up duration.

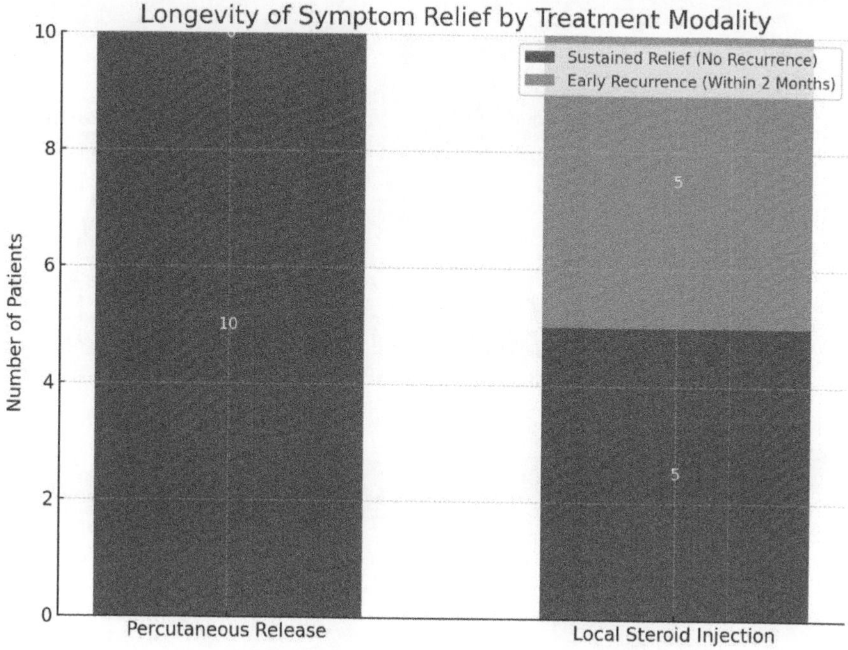

Figure 2.8. *Longevity of symptom relief, within follow-up period, per treatment modality*

2.10.9. *Tendon release assessment in the PR group*

Intraoperative findings among the ten patients who underwent percutaneous A1 pulley release revealed complete tendon release in seven cases (70%) and partial release in three cases (30%).

Release was confirmed by the disappearance of grating resistance and free gliding of the tendon on flexion-extension testing. While a one-tailed binomial test ($P = 0.17$) did not give a statistically significant P-value < 0.05, the trend favored complete release outcomes.

No conversions to open surgery or neurovascular complications were observed, reinforcing the safety as well as the efficacy of the percutaneous technique in achieving adequate tendon decompression.

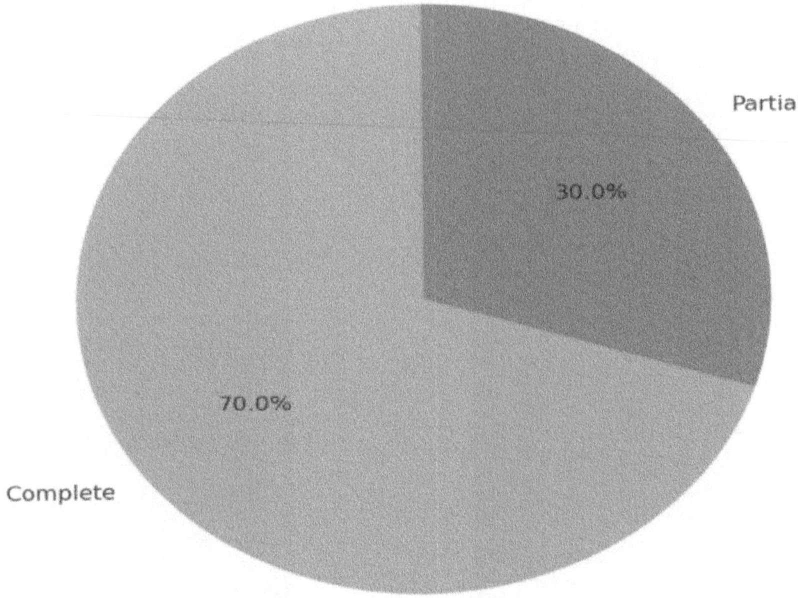

Figure 2.9. *Intraoperative tendon release assessment in percutaneous release group*

2.11. Complications

2.11.1. *Tendon/neurovascular bundle injury*

In our study, we monitored for incidence of any neurovascular complications following treatment for trigger digits. The evaluation across both modalities showed no cases of neurovascular injury reported in either treatment group. A chi-square test was used to assess the statistical significance of this observation, yielding a chi-square value of 0.0 (df = 0) and a P-value of 1.0. This showed that the incidence of neurovascular injuries did not differ significantly between the two techniques.

The lack of any complications in the two groups shows that an LSI, as well as PR when carried out with a proper technique and anatomical accuracy, is safe with regard to neurovascular integrity. The results support the safety indications of PR, even on the basis of previous anatomical issues so long as the procedure takes the existing surface landmarks and precautions.

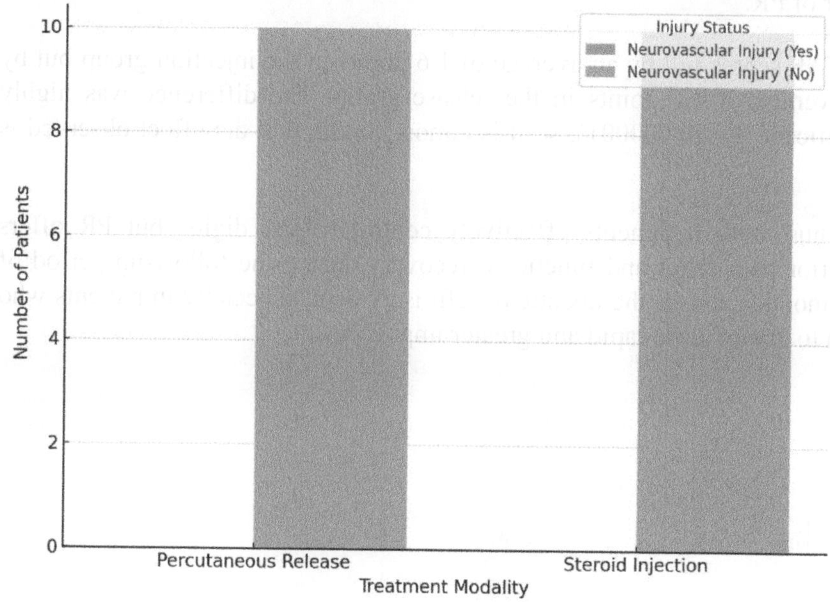

Figure 2.10. *Comparison of tendon/neurovascular bundle injury incidence by treatment modality*

2.11.2. *Infection rate*

This finding establishes a safety for both modalities, provided strict aseptic techniques are followed, strict technique is applied, and strict postoperative care is provided. It also supports existing literature, which states that local corticosteroid injection and percutaneous A1 pulley release are well-tolerated, minimally invasive procedures with a low risk of iatrogenic infection in appropriately selected patients.

2.11.3. *Post-treatment functional outcome assessment*

Functional outcomes were assessed using the DASH score and the VAS pain score, both pre-operatively and two months post-operatively, and the results were compared between the LSI and PR.

The improvement in score for the LSI group was 12.5 DASH points on average, and for the PR group, 23.7 points. A P-value of 0.003 by independent t-test showed a positive statistically significant difference in favor of PR.

VAS scores fell by an average of 1.6 points in the injection group but by an average of 4.6 points in the release group. The difference was highly significant (P < 0.000001), so it is almost certain that the effect observed is real.

Thus, both treatments effectively control trigger digits, but PR offers superior pain relief and functional recovery during the follow-up period of two months, and its therapeutic benefit is evident, especially in patients who wish to obtain more rapid and greater improvement.

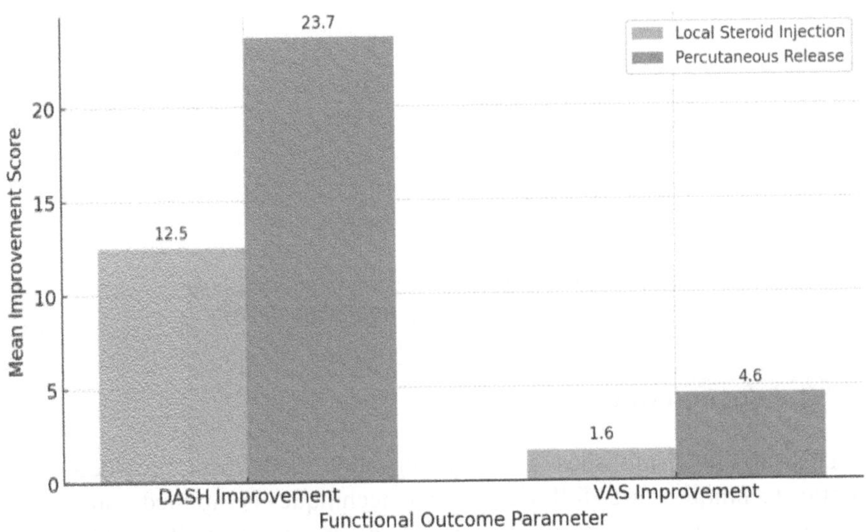

Figure 2.11. *Comparison of post-treatment functional outcome assessment*

2.12. Discussion

Trigger digit is a common hand condition that affects the function and quality of life associated with the hand, especially in middle and older adults. This is a prospective comparative study of LSI and percutaneous A1 pulley release in terms of functional results, pain relief, recurrence and complications (White and Sampson 2021).

Both treatments resulted in initial relief of symptoms, but PR always had the better short-term results. Patients who received release had more significant improvement in DASH and VAS scores, demonstrating improved functional recovery and pain relief (Yavari et al. 2023). These findings support research from the past that emphasizes the mechanical nature of trigger digit. Definitive division of the hypertrophied A1 pulley provides tendon gliding restoration while providing a long-term symptom solution, whereas steroid injections only provide transient anti-inflammatories and do not resolve the underlying anatomical constriction, explaining the increased recurrence rate seen with injections.

Recurrence was much higher following steroid injection, and approximately one-half of the patients had a return of symptoms within two months. No recurrences occurred among the PR group, as shown in previous studies of higher recurrence rates after corticosteroid treatment, especially for patients with a long duration of symptoms or systemic comorbidities (Bhat et al. 2023).

Both modalities had an excellent safety profile, with no nerve vascular injuries or infections reported. However, the study suffered from a small sample size and a short follow-up period, but the evidence still supports percutaneous A1 pulley release as a more effective and long-lasting option in more moderate-to-severe or recurrent cases of the condition.

2.13. Conclusion

PR was better than steroid injection in terms of pain relief, functional recovery and durability and recurrence prevention. Both approaches were safe, but recurrence rates of injections were higher, which limits the long-term efficacy of this therapy. Being a direct way of correcting the pathology of the A1 pulley, PR provides a definitive and lasting solution, particularly in cases that are moderate to severe or recurrent. Therefore, percutaneous A1 pulley release is advocated as the treatment of choice, with decisions made on an individual basis, based on severity of symptoms, comorbidities and functional demands.

2.14. References

Bhat, A.K., Vyas, R., Acharya, A.M., Rajagopal, K.V. (2023). De Quervain's tenosynovitis: A non-randomized two-armed study comparing ultrasound-guided steroid injection with surgical release. *Musculoskeletal Surgery*, 107(1), 105–114.

Changhez, J., James, S., Jamala, F., Khan, S., Khan, M.Z., Gul, S., Zainab, I. (2024). Evaluating the efficacy and accuracy of AI-assisted diagnostic techniques in endometrial carcinoma: A systematic review. *Cureus*, 16(5), e60973. doi: 10.7759/cureus.60973.

Chanthanapodi, P. and Aodsup, S. (2025). Comparative results of percutaneous and open surgery for trigger fingers: A propensity score analysis. *Frontiers in Surgery*, 12, 1509292.

Ciarambino, T., Crispino, P., Leto, G., Mastrolorenzo, E., Para, O., Giordano, M. (2022). Influence of gender in diabetes mellitus and its complication. *International Journal of Molecular Sciences*, 23(16), 8850.

Freedman, B.R., Mooney, D.J., Weber, E. (2022). Advances toward transformative therapies for tendon diseases. *Science Translational Medicine*, 14(661), eabl8814.

Hollins, A.W., Hein, R., Atia, A., Taskindoust, M., Darner, G., Shammas, R., Mithani, S.K. (2022). Symptom duration and diabetic control influence success of steroid injection in trigger finger. *Plastic and Reconstructive Surgery*, 150(2), 357e–63e.

Karki, M., Sharma, R., Sunuwar, D.R., Gupta, R.S., Singh, D.R., Lama, S., Bhandari, K.K., Tamang, R.K., Chaudhary, N.K. (2025). Effect of percutaneous release versus steroid injection among adults with trigger fingers: A randomized clinical trial. *BMC Musculoskeletal Disorders*, 26(1), 1.

Kissin, E. (2024). Ultrasonography of the hand and wrist. In *Clinical Atlas of Musculoskeletal Ultrasound in Rheumatology*, Yinh, J., Kissin, E., DeMarco, P.J., Kohler, M.J. (eds). Springer, Cham, 195–239.

Kumar, A., Batta, P., Ahuja, S., Rathore, P.S. (eds) (2026). *AI-driven Innovations in Physiotherapy and Oncology 1*. ISTE Ltd, London and Wiley, Hoboken, NJ.

Lalehzarian, S.P., Gowd, A.K., Liu, J.N. (2021). Machine learning in orthopaedic surgery. *World Journal of Orthopedics*, 12(9), 685.

Levine, N., Young, C., Allen, I., Immerman, I. (2022). Percutaneous release of trigger finger with and without steroid injection: A systematic review and meta-analysis. *Bulletin of the Hospital for Joint Diseases*, 80(2), 137–144.

Ng, N.Y., Sirisena, R., Chua, Y.X. (2023). Management of stenosing flexor tenosynovitis in primary care. *Singapore Medical Journal*, 64(4), 255–261.

Pathak, S.K., Salunke, A.A., Menon, P.H., Thivari, P., Nandy, K., Yongsheng, C.H. (2022). Corticosteroid injection for the treatment of trigger finger: A meta-analysis of randomised control trials. *The Journal of Hand Surgery (Asian-Pacific Volume)*, 27(01), 89–97.

Patrinely, J.R. Jr., Johnson, S.P., Drolet, B.C. (2021). Trigger finger corticosteroid injection with and without local anesthetic: A randomized, double-blind controlled trial. *Hand*, 16(5), 619–623.

Sayed, D., Abd-Elsayed, A., Falowski, S., Deer, T., Sagarwala, S., Kim, B.Y., Kim, D.H. (2024). Surgican instruments. In *Minimally Invasive Surgical Procedures for Pain*, Sayed, D., Abd-Elsayed, A., Falowski, S., Deer, T. (eds). Oxford Academic, New York, 9–24.

Schmitt, R., Hesse, N., Grunz, J.P. (2022). Tendons and tendon sheaths of the hand: An update on MRI. *RöFo-Fortschritte auf dem Gebiet der Röntgenstrahlen und der bildgebenden Verfahren*, 194(12), 1307–1321.

Stone, S., Malanga, G.A., Capella, T. (2021). Corticosteroids: Review of the history, the effectiveness, and adverse effects in the treatment of joint pain. *Pain Physician*, 24(S1), S233.

Vogt, B., Lueckingsmeier, M., Gosheger, G., Laufer, A., Toporowski, G., Antfang, C., Roedl, R., Frommer, A. (2024). Magnetically driven antegrade intramedullary lengthening nails for tibial lengthening: Evaluation of 67 treatments. *The Bone & Joint Journal*, 106(3), 293–302.

White, R.Z. and Sampson, M.J. (2021). Assessment of short-term response and review of technique of ultrasound-guided percutaneous A1 pulley release for the treatment of trigger finger. *Journal of Medical Imaging and Radiation Oncology*, 65(6), 672–677.

Yavari, M., Modaresi, S.M., Hassanpour, S.E., Moosavizadeh, S.M., Tabrizi, A. (2023). Clinical study between percutaneous ultrasound-guided release and open classic surgery in treating multiple trigger fingers. *Advanced Biomedical Research*, 12(1), 88.

Zorzi, A.R. (ed.) (2024). *Advancements in Synovial Joint Science-Structure, Function, and Beyond*. IntechOpen, London.

3

Rigid Versus Hybrid Fixation in Both-Bone Forearm Fractures: An AI-Supported Comparative Study

Both of these are complex injuries, including radius and ulna fractures (bones of the forearm). Open reduction and internal fixation (ORI) with plating has long been considered the gold standard solution; however, a less invasive option is hybrid fixation – ulnar intramedullary nailing and radial plating in combination. This is an artificial intelligence (AI)-supported, comparative study of clinical, radiological and functional outcomes of rigid plating versus hybrid fixation for adult diaphyseal both-bone forearm fractures. A prospective cohort of 48 patients was divided up into two groups: rigid fixation (plating of both bones) and hybrid fixation (ulnar IM nailing with radial plating). Outcomes measured were time to union, union rates, postoperative mobilization, complication rate and functional recovery as measured by the Anderson scoring system. An objective comparison between these parameters was provided by AI-assisted analysis. The outcomes of the hybrid group were faster union, reduced malunion, better functionality and range of motion, less postoperative pain and rehabilitation requirements and no increase in complications. The results of this study indicate that using hybrid fixation offers biomechanical and functional advantages in selected patients. The clinical evaluation with the help of AI helps the clinical decision-making support for individualized fixation strategies. Hybrid fixation may therefore be a suitable alternative to rigid plating for appropriately selected both-bone forearm fractures.

3.1. Introduction

Both-bone forearm fracture (diaphysis of the radius and ulna) is among the most challenging injuries to treat in orthopedic trauma (Rafi and Tiwari 2023).

Chapter written by Manthena Ramakrishna Vittal VERMA and Paresh V. PATIL.

For a color version of all the figures in this chapter, see www.iste.co.uk/kumar/orthopedic1.zip.

The forearm is a biomechanical unit that permits pronation and supination, which is required daily for positioning the hand. Even mild malalignment, rotational deformity or shortening of either bone may reduce utilization of the upper limb to a large extent. Therefore, treatment goals are anatomical reduction, stable fixation, early mobilization and restoration of forearm rotation (Caruso et al. 2021).

Historically, conservative treatment with closed reduction and casting had an overall tendency toward malunion, non-union and poor function, particularly in adults. The introduction of open reduction and internal fixation (ORIF) with plate osteosynthesis revolutionized the treatment of forearm fractures by enabling the precise anatomical restoration of the fracture and providing rigid stability (Bhoir 2022). Plating of both radius and ulna has proven to have high union rates and predictable functional recovery and is therefore the gold standard for treating adult diaphyseal forearm fractures.

Effective, rigid plating for both the bones has its disadvantages: extensive soft tissue dissection, longer surgery, increased risk of infection, neurovascular injury and periosteal stripping, which can ruin biology and delay healing (Shafiq et al. 2021). These problems have led to the development of less invasive techniques that allow soft tissue conservation with adequate mechanical stability.

Intramedullary nailing (IMN) offers a minimally invasive alternative, particularly for the ulna, which has a relatively straight medullary canal and subcutaneous location. IMN helps in minimizing periosteal disruption and exposure and may help in faster healing (Bleakley 2024). However, IMN alone can offer poor rotational stability and alignment control than plating, and especially it is poor in complicated fractures. Hybrid fixation – nailing the ulna and plating of the radius – has been created to combine biomechanical benefits with biological preservation (Huxman et al. 2025).

Recent studies have suggested hybrid fixation is comparable to or better than rigid plating in certain instances of broken bone, with the benefit of quicker union, improved functional outcome, less stiffness after surgery and less complication rates. Nonetheless, results from the literature are mixed, and there is still no consensus on the desired optimal strategy. Traditional analyses have often been based on modestly sized data sets and may therefore miss potentially clinically significant patterns.

Artificial intelligence (AI)-assisted data analysis in orthopedic research can aid in presenting more objective multidimensional evaluations of outcomes (Tariq et al. 2023). "AI is promoting pattern recognition in demographic, clinical, radiological and functional variables to write evidence-based decision making and personalised treatment strategies" (Gorelik et al. 2020).

The aim of this study is to compare the outcomes following rigid plating and hybrid fixation in both-bone forearm fractures. Objectives include the assessment of differences in postoperative mobilization, union time and rates, complication rates, functional outcome using the Anderson scoring system and establishing whether the hybrid fixation will have comparable or superior results in adult diaphyseal forearm fractures.

3.2. Literature review

Both-bone forearm fractures of the long bones are complex in their anatomy and also biomechanics. The integrity of the function of the forearm depends on the proper restoration of the length, alignment, rotation and radial bow to allow the function of pronation and supination. Inadequate treatment may result in malunion, non-united fractures and restricted motion with long-term disability, and surgical fixation is the standard treatment in adults.

3.2.1. *Evolution of forearm fracture management*

Historically, conservative treatment with closed reduction and casting resulted in high rates of malunion, as was reported by Schatzker, the AO group, Bohler and Charnley, all of whom emphasized the failure of non-operative management in adults (Kumar et al. 2025). Bohler emphasized the difficulty in maintaining length and alignment with traction alone, while Charnley strongly advocated operative management as the treatment of choice for adult forearm fractures.

Advances in radiography and implant design ultimately made ORIF well-known. Compression plating offered the advantages of anatomical reduction, rigid fixation, early mobilization and better union and functional results (Bhoir 2022).

3.2.2. *Rigid fixation using plate osteosynthesis*

Plate fixation of both is the standard of care in diaphyseal fracture for radius and ulna. Dynamic compression plates (DCP), limited-contact DCP (LC-DCP) and locking compression plates (LCPs) provide rigid stability and great rotational control (Shevate et al. 2022). Anderson directly associated favorable functional results with anatomical reduction with plating.

Multiple studies include dual plating report rates of union >90–95% and restored forearm rotation. Schemitsch and Richards highlighted the significance of restoring the radial bow, as it plays a crucial role in maintaining optimal grip strength and forearm rotational movements. However, rigid plating still requires extensive soft tissue dissection, higher operative time, blood loss, risks of infection, neurovascular damage and irritation of the soft tissues surrounding the implants (Marchand et al. 2021).

3.2.3. *IMN of forearm bones*

Intramedullary fixation has been investigated for over 100 years since wire fixation and pin techniques were first developed. Kuntscher introduced long-last nails that provided axial stability without opening up of the fracture site (Bekos et al. 2021). Innovators that came later – Rush, Sage, Talwalkar, etc. – perfected nail designs in order to introduce rotational stability.

Early intramedullary methods of treatment for forearm fractures were riddled with high rates of non-union and malalignment, which were mostly due to the lack of rotational control. Non-union was reported by Smith and Sage in up to 38% of cases with wire fixation. Improvements such as square nails, elastic nails and interlocking intramedullary nails reduced non-union and surgical morbidity.

3.2.4. *Hybrid fixation: concept and rationale*

Hybrid fixation combines two techniques: a plate is used to fix the radius, and an intramedullary nail is used to stabilize the ulna. This technique allows knowledge of the anatomical alignment of the radial plate and the ulna's minimally invasive, subcutaneous nailing with less soft-tissue damage.

Use of hybrid fixation provides strong biomechanical stability, reduced complications and improved functional results compared to isolated nailing or plating. Lee et al. reported that the advantages of hybrid fixation are a combination of rotational stability provided by the radial plate and the biologic effects of ulnar intramedullary fixation, particularly for simple fractures – mid-shaft ulnar fractures.

3.2.5. *Comparative studies: rigid versus hybrid fixation*

Several comparative studies have compared rigid fixation and hybrid techniques. Locked IMN and plating resulted in similar functional results; however, locked IMN resulted in a shorter operative time and less blood loss.

Seo et al. (2022) suggested slightly superior outcomes of dual plating, but it was seen that the hybrid fixation was useful for those fractures that could not be plated alone.

The hybrid fixation technique has similar union rates and functional scores while reducing surgical time and soft tissue complications. Hopf et al. (2020) stated that, despite differences in torsional stability as compared with plating, intramedullary fixation offers the advantage of preservation of biology and rapid healing of the periosteum.

3.2.6. *Functional outcomes and complications*

Functional outcomes after fixation of fracture of the forearm are usually measured as Anderson scores, range of movement, grip strength and pain levels. The literature is consistent in stating that anatomic reduction and early mobilization are crucial to success. Hybrid fixation has been associated with a more rapid recovery as well as reduced postoperative stiffness in selected cases (Deng et al. 2021).

Complication profiles vary. Rigid fixation may lead to infection, implant protrusion or soft tissue damage. Hybrid fixation might be related to implant migration or poorer rotational control with some fracture patterns (Thakur 2022).

Overall, the majority of studies demonstrate either similar rates of complications or lower rates of complications with the use of hybrid fixation when patients are properly selected for this treatment option.

3.2.7. *Role of advanced and AI-assisted analysis*

Modern orthopedics focuses on using data in decision-making to optimize treatment decisions.

AI-aided analysis of comparative data: AI provides for the objective assessment of demographics, fracture patterns, union times and functional scores, and complications and thus enhances the prediction of outcomes and facilitates the provision of personalized care (Kutbi 2024).

3.3. Materials and methods

Study design: this is a prospective, comparative study conducted at Krishna Hospital and Medical Research Centre, Karad, under the Department of Orthopedics. The study compares the outcomes of both-bone forearm fractures treated with rigid fixation (plating of both radius and ulna) and hybrid fixation (plating of the radius and IMN of the ulna).

3.3.1. *Duration of study*

Data collection period: 18 months (March 2023 to September 2024).

Data analysis period: 6 months (October 2024 to May 2025).

3.3.2. *Ethical approval*

Approval was obtained from the Institutional Ethical Committee (IEC) before the initiation of the study.

Informed written consent was obtained from all participants.

3.3.3. *Study population*

Patients presenting with both-bone forearm fractures (radius and ulna shaft fractures) at Krishna Hospital, Karad, were assessed for inclusion.

3.3.4. *Inclusion criteria*

History of specific trauma.

Radiographically confirmed diaphyseal fracture of both radius and ulna.

Age >18 years.

No history of previous forearm trauma.

Patients undergoing rigid fixation (plating of both bones) or hybrid fixation (IM nailing of ulna + plating of radius).

Both male and female patients.

3.3.4.1. *Exclusion criteria*

Open mid-shaft fractures.

Pathological fractures.

Fractures with associated vascular or nerve injuries.

Osteoporotic bones.

Associated humeral condyle or wrist fractures.

Monteggia and Galeazzi fractures and their variants.

3.3.5. *Sample size*

Total sample size: 48 patients.

Divided into two groups of 24 patients each:

– *Group 1*: Rigid fixation (plate fixation of radius and ulna).

– *Group 2*: Hybrid fixation (plate fixation of radius and IMN of ulna).

Sample size calculated using a standard statistical formula based on prior outcomes (52.4% versus 87%).

Formula used:

$$n = \frac{(p_1 q_1 + p_2 q_2) \times (Z_{1-\alpha} + Z_{1-\beta})^2}{(p_1 - p_2)^2}$$

where:

– $p_1 = 0.524$, $q_1 = 1 - p_1 = 0.476$;

– $p_2 = 0.87$, $q_2 = 1 - p_2 = 0.13$;

– $Z_{1-\alpha/2} = 1.96$ (for 95% confidence);

– $Z_{1-\beta} = 0.84$ (for 80% power);

– $(p_1 - p_2)^2 = (0.524 - 0.87)^2 = 0.1204$.

Calculation (simplified explanation):

$$n = \frac{(0.524 \times 0.476 + 0.87 \times 0.13) \times (1.96 + 0.84)^2}{(0.346)^2}$$

$$n = \frac{(0.249 + 0.1131) \times 7.84}{0.1197}$$

$$n = \frac{0.3621 \times 7.84}{0.1197} = \frac{2.84}{0.1197} \approx 23.7$$

So, each group requires approximately 24 participants, making the total sample size 48 patients.

3.3.5.1. *Grouping and randomization*

Patients were randomly allocated into two groups after applying inclusion/exclusion criteria.

Informed consent was taken prior to allocation.

3.3.6. *Observation and results*

Both-bone forearm fractures (fractures of the radius and ulna) are common orthopedic injuries that often require surgical intervention to restore function and alignment. The two primary surgical approaches are as follows:

1) Rigid fixation (plate fixation of radius and ulna): both bones are fixed with compression plates and screws.

2) Hybrid fixation (plate fixation of radius + IMN of ulna): the radius is plated, while the ulna is stabilized with an intramedullary nail.

This study compares the results of these two methods of fixation in terms of union rates, functional recovery, complications and patient satisfaction.

The study was done on 48 patients, 24 in each group. In the rigid fixation group, 45.8% were aged between 30 and 50 years, 41.7% were older than 50 years and 12.5% were younger than 30 years.

Group 2 (hybrid fixation) had a similar distribution, with 41.7% in both the 30–50 and >50 age groups and 16.7% aged <30. The difference in age distribution between groups was not statistically significant ($P > 0.05$).

The study included an equal number of males and females in Group 1 (rigid fixation) (50% each), while Group 2 (hybrid fixation) had a higher proportion of males (62.5%) compared to females (37.5%). However, this difference in gender distribution between the two groups was not statistically significant ($P > 0.05$).

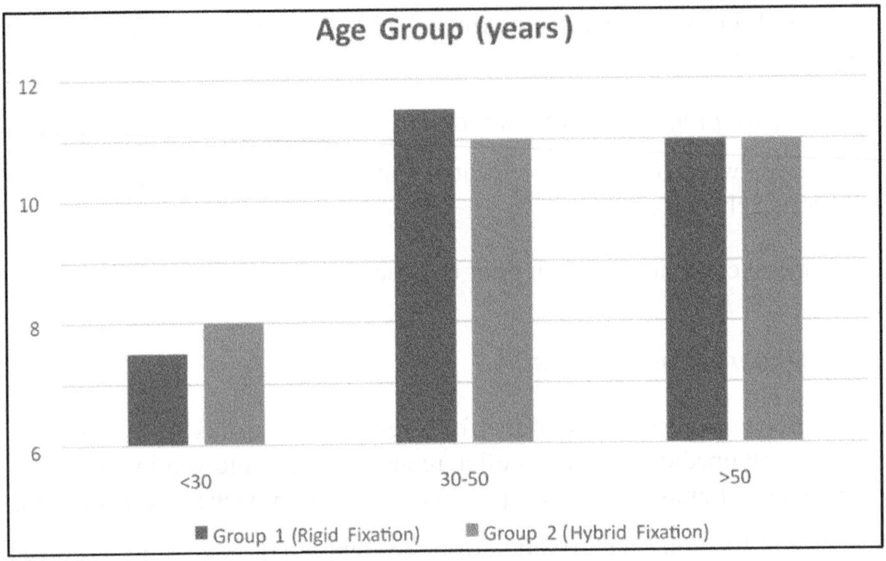

Figure 3.1. *Distribution of age of the patients in rigid fixation and hybrid fixation groups*

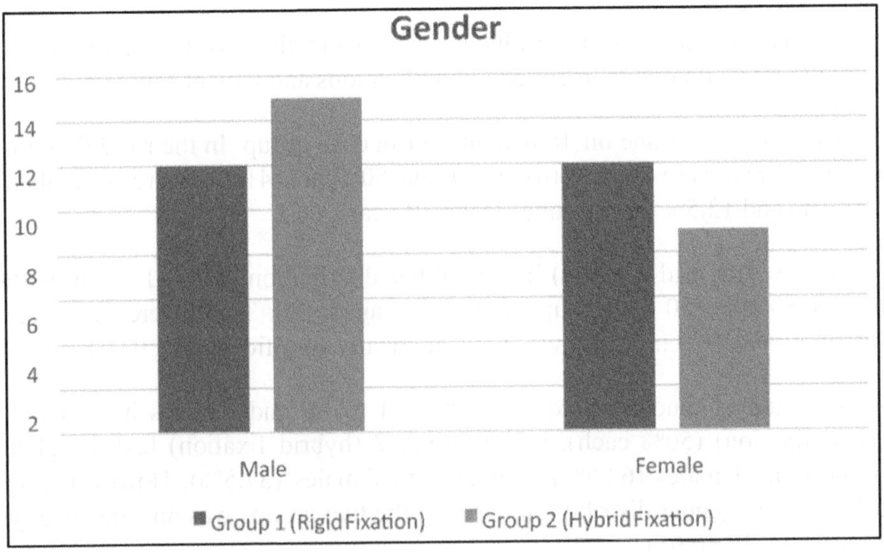

Figure 3.2. *Gender distribution of patients in rigid fixation versus hybrid fixation groups*

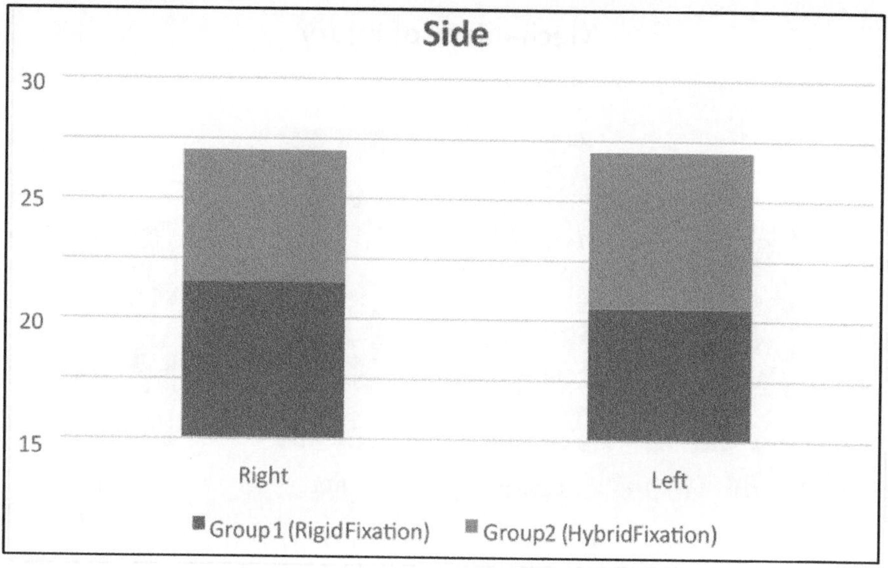

Figure 3.3. *Distribution of affected side in rigid fixation versus hybrid fixation groups*

The laterality of forearm fractures was similarly distributed between the two treatment groups. In Group 1 (rigid fixation), 54.2% of fractures involved the right side, while 45.8% involved the left. The hybrid fixation group had a nearly reversed age skewness of 45.8% of the population in the 30–50 age range, 41.7% older than 50 age range and 12.5% younger than 30 age range. The distribution was not statistically significant ($P > 0.05$).

There were similar injury mechanisms among both groups. Road traffic accidents accounted for 29.2% and 29.2% in both groups, and assaults made up 29.2% in the rigid group and 25% in the hybrid group. Falls and sports injuries accounted for 20.8–25% of cases each. No significant differences were determined ($P > 0.05$).

Distal fractures were the most common fractures in both groups (50% in the rigid group and 41.6% in the hybrid group). Mid-shaft fracture was next (33.3 versus 37.5), and proximal fractures were least common (16.6 versus 20.8). Location difference in distribution was not statistically significant ($P > 0.05$).

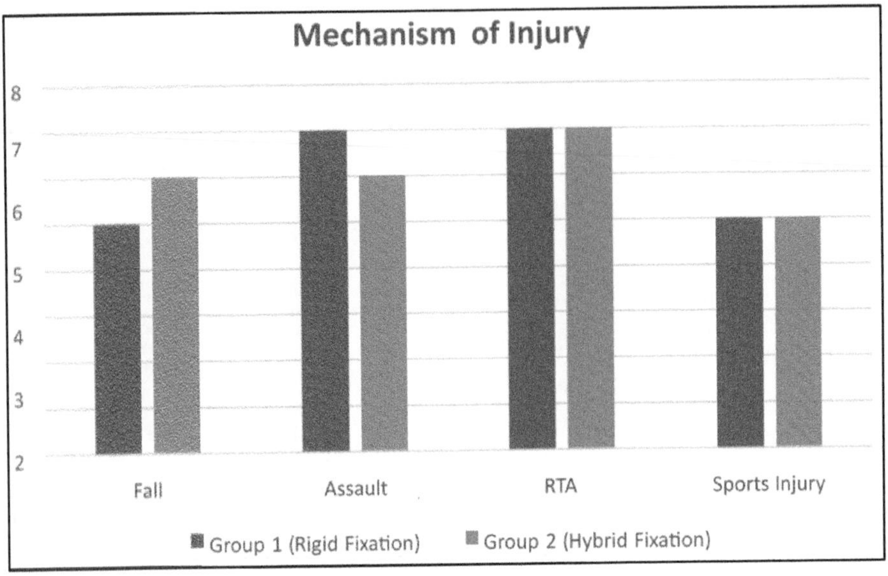

Figure 3.4. *Distribution of mechanism of injury in rigid fixation and hybrid fixation groups*

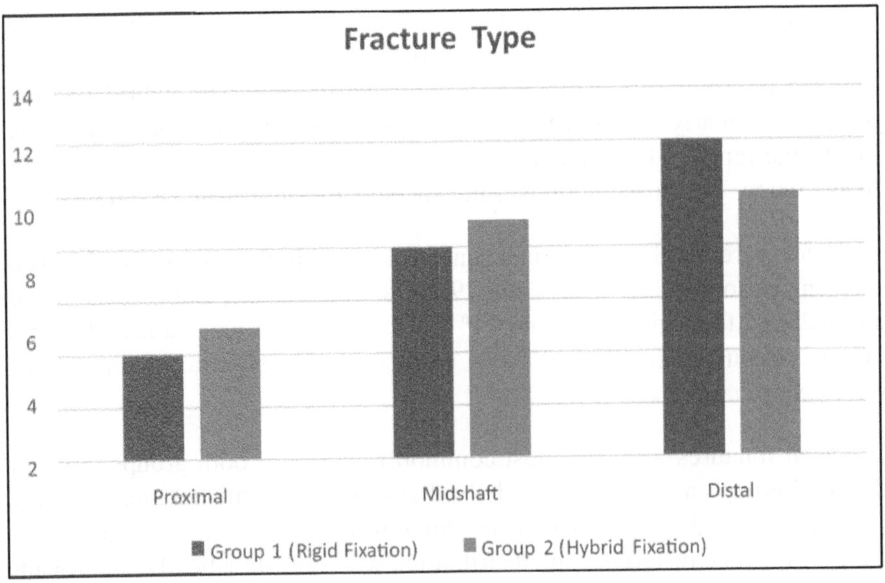

Figure 3.5. *Location of fracture distribution in rigid fixation versus hybrid fixation groups*

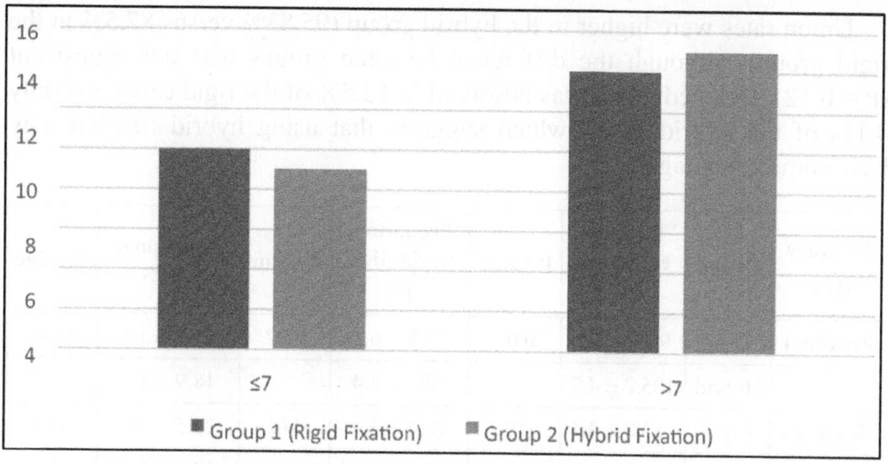

Figure 3.6. *Time to surgical intervention with rigid fixation (in days) versus hybrid fixation groups*

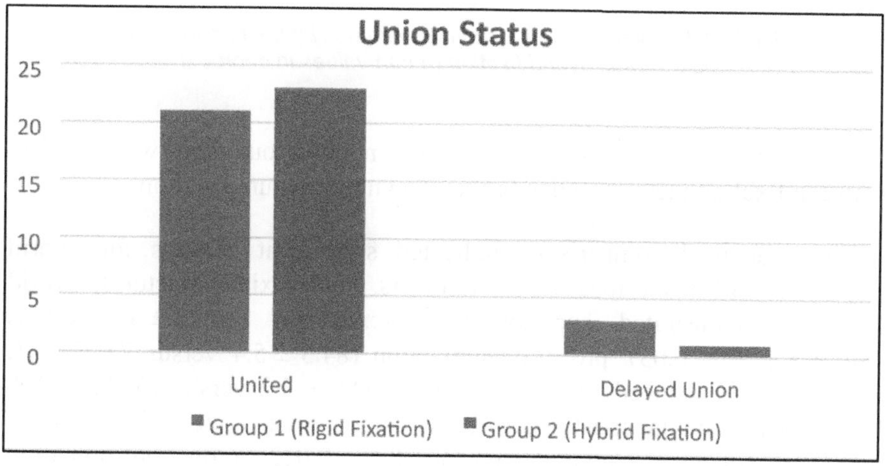

Figure 3.7. *Fracture union result in rigid fixation and hybrid fixation groups*

Timing for surgery was similar for both approaches. Most of the patients in both groups underwent surgery after seven days (58.3% versus 62.5%). Early intervention (seven or less days) was in 41.7% of rigid cases and 37.5% of hybrid cases. The difference in timing was not significant ($P > 0.05$).

Union rates were higher in the hybrid group (95.83% versus 87.5% in the rigid group), although the difference between groups was not significant (P = 0.12). Delayed union was observed in 12.5% of the rigid cases and only 4.1% of the hybrid cases, which suggests that using hybrid fixation may have some advantage.

Fracture type	**Group**	**Flexion/ extension (°)**	**P-value**	**Pronation/ supination (°)**	**P-value**	**Functional loss (%)**	**P-value**
Proximal	Rigid	98.6 ± 5.2	0.03	73.2 ± 6.1	0.02	23.1 ± 3.8	0.04
	Hybrid	105.2 ± 4.7		84.3 ± 5.4		18.9 ± 3.2	
Mid-shaft	Rigid	113.8 ± 4.1	0.012	76.7 ± 5.3	0.02	22.5 ± 2.9	0.01
	Hybrid	117.5 ± 3.8		83.3 ± 4.9		19.3 ± 2.7	
Distal	Rigid	119.4 ± 3.5	0.009	79.2 ± 4.7	0.04	18.7 ± 2.5	0.007
	Hybrid	121.9 ± 3.2		84.3 ± 4.2		16.4 ± 2.1	

Table 3.1. *Comparative functional outcomes by fracture location: rigid versus hybrid fixation (mean values in degrees)*

A significant difference (P < 0.05) in functional outcomes was noted in between fixation methods when broken down by fracture location.

The statistical comparisons indicated significant benefits for hybrid fixation for all of the measured parameters. For proximal fractures, hybrid fixation demonstrated superior flexion/extension (105.2°± 4.7 versus 98.6°± 5.2, P = 0.03), pronation/supination (84.3°± 5.4 versus 73.2°± 6.1, P = 0.02) and reduced functional loss (18.9% ± 3.2 versus 23.1% ± 3.8, P = 0.04). Simultaneously significant improvements were displayed in mid-shaft fractures (flexion/extension P = 0.012, pronation/supination P = 0.02) as well as in distal fractures (flexion/extension P = 0.009, pronation/supination P = 0.04). The highest functional gain was observed in distal fractures, with lower functional loss in the hybrid fixation group (16.4 ± 2.1) compared to the comparison group (18.7 ± 2.5), which was statistically significant (P = 0.007). With consistent results, it is proposed that hybrid fixation has biomechanical advantages that translate to improved functional results irrespective of fracture location.

Using the Anderson score, we found a significant difference (P = 0.05) in functional outcomes. For distal fractures, the results for hybrid fixation were better (64 versus 50 good results; P = 0.02). Both proximal and mid-shaft fractures had similar excellent/good rates, but hybrid fixation abolished poor outcomes in mid-shaft fractures (0 versus 5%; 0 versus 5%; P = 0.04) and reduced poor outcomes in proximal fractures (5 versus 10%; P = 0.04). The results of this study suggest that hybrid fixation has important clinical benefits, particularly for distal fractures.

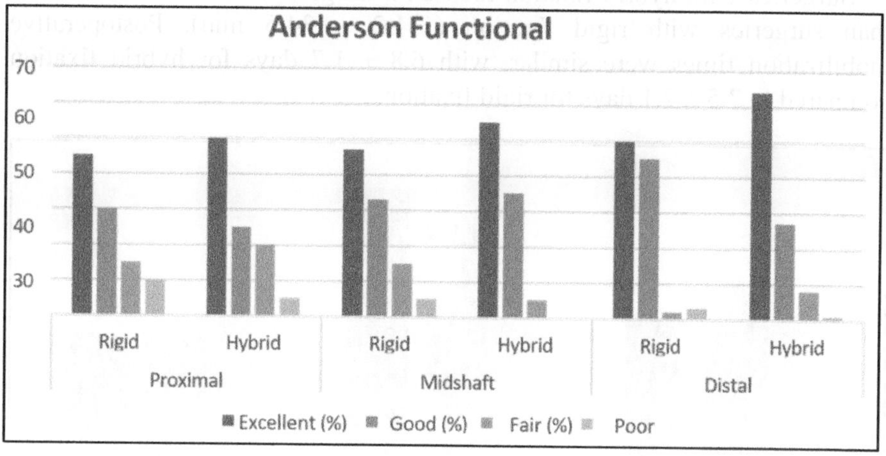

Figure 3.8. *Anderson functional score distribution by fracture type and fixation method*

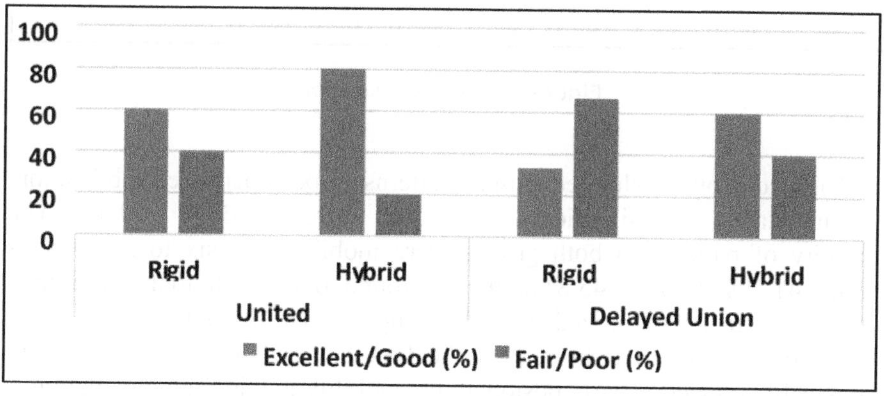

Figure 3.9. *Relationship between union status and functional outcomes (Anderson Score)*

There was a significant relationship (P < 0.05) between fracture union and function. Hybrid fixation led to a greater excellent/good rate (80 versus 60% for rigid; P = 0.01) in united fractures. Even with the delayed unions, the hybrid fixation still performed better than the rigid (60 versus 33.3%; P = 0.03). Non-unions had poor functional scores in both methods, although the small sample size did not allow a statistical difference (P > 0.05). Therefore, hybrid fixation enhances union as well as functional recovery.

Surgeries with hybrid fixation took on average 118.6 ± 29.8 min shorter than surgeries with rigid fixation (131.2 ± 34.5 min). Postoperative mobilization times were similar, with 6.8 ± 1.7 days for hybrid fixation compared to 7.5 ± 2.1 days for rigid fixation.

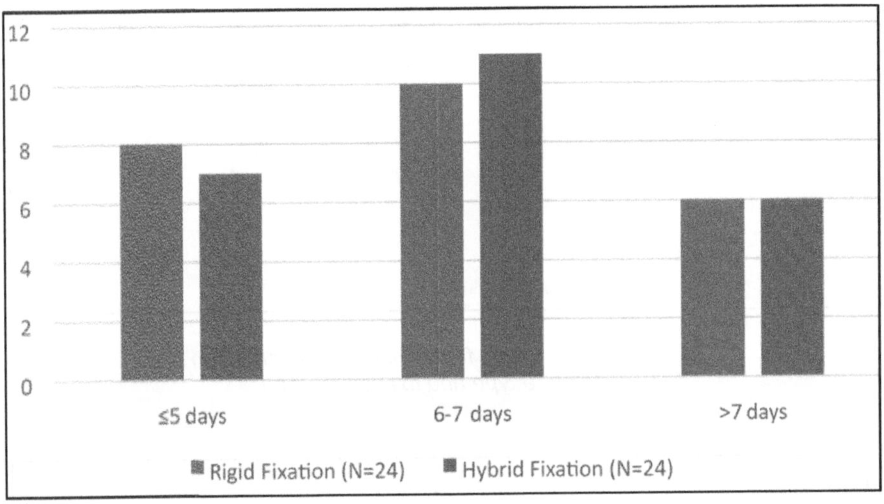

Figure 3.10. *Mobilization time*

The two groups exhibited similar patterns of postoperative mobilization, and no statistically significant differences were found (P > 0.05). The majority of patients in both groups were mobilized in six to seven days (rigid: 41.7%; hybrid: 45.8%), while around one-fourth took more than seven days to be mobilized in each group (25.0% for both). The similar distribution seems to indicate that the fixation method does not have an appreciable impact on early postoperative mobility in this study population.

Hybrid fixation resulted in faster union (5 weeks versus 7 weeks, P = 0.02) of united fractures. In delayed unions, the healing was slightly slower with hybrid fixation (8 weeks versus 5 weeks; P = 0.11). However overall, the average union time was shorter with hybrid fixation (8.9 ± 2.7 weeks) than with rigid fixation (10.4 ± 3.2 weeks; P = 0.03), reporting a potential positive effect on fracture healing. More studies are required with a focus on delayed unions.

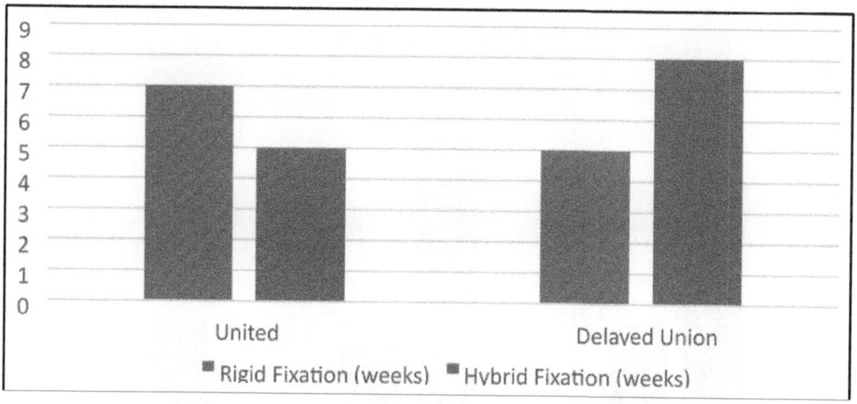

Figure 3.11. *Comparative fracture union times between rigid and hybrid fixation methods*

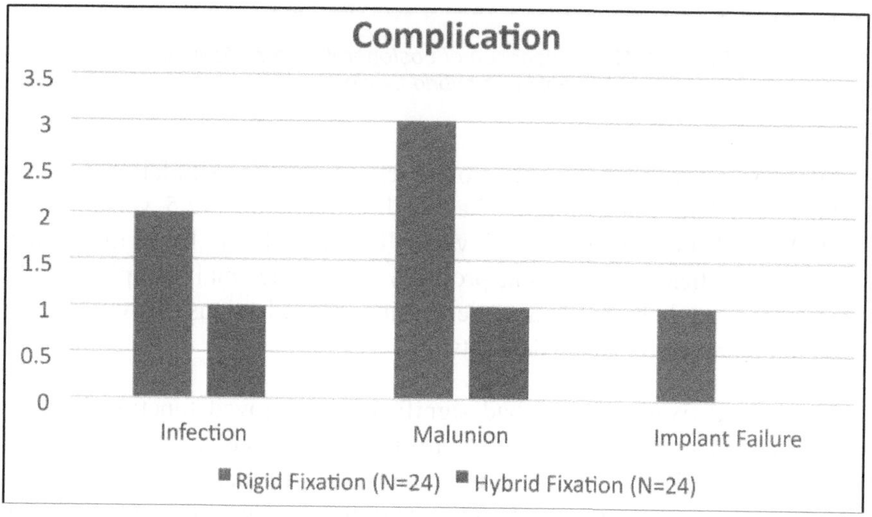

Figure 3.12. *Comparative fracture union times between rigid and hybrid fixation methods*

The study compared union times between rigid and hybrid fixation methods, revealing that hybrid fixation achieved faster union (5 weeks versus 7 weeks, P = 0.02) in united cases, while delayed unions trended towards longer healing with hybrid fixation (8 weeks versus 5 weeks, P = 0.11). Overall, hybrid fixation demonstrated a significantly shorter mean union time (8.9 ± 2.7 weeks) compared to rigid fixation (10.4 ± 3.2 weeks, P = 0.03), suggesting its potential advantage in accelerating fracture healing.

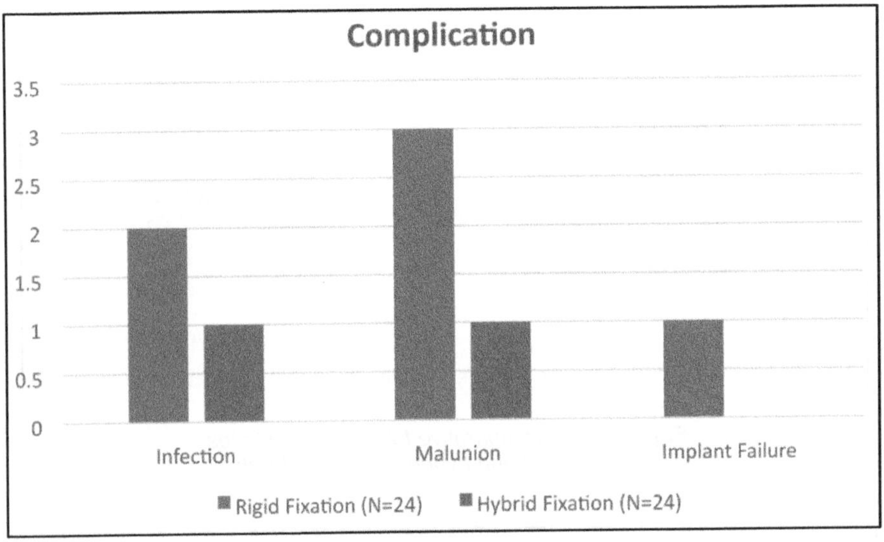

Figure 3.13. *Comparison of postoperative complications between rigid and hybrid fixation techniques*

Infection rates in 24 patients from each group were similar (8.3 versus 4.2%; P = 1.00). Rigid fixation had higher malunion (12.5 versus 4.2%; P = 0.03) and implant failure (4.2 versus 0%; P = 0.31). These differences were not statistically significant, probably due to the small sample, but the trend is toward hybrid fixation decreasing complications. However, this needs to be proven on larger data sets.

The hybrid fixation group had significantly improved functional results with an excellent/good Anderson score in 58.3% versus 41.7% in the rigid fixation group (P = 0.04). Excellent individual results were higher with hybrid fixation (25.0 versus 16.7%), and the greatest improvement was reducing poor outcomes (16.7 versus 25.0%). It is proven that hybrid fixation results in better functional recovery without increasing suboptimal results.

Patients treated with hybrid fixation had significantly less pain at every follow-up interval. The difference was greatest at six weeks (50% versus 75%; P = 0.03) and six months (8.3% versus 25%; P = 0.02). Pain resolution trends favored hybrid fixation at three months (20.8% versus 41.7%; P = 0.04), whereas the difference between groups at 2.5 months (33.3% versus 58.3%; P = 0.06) showed an impressive trend but did not reach significance for analysis.

Overall, the development of hybrid fixation is conducive to accelerating and achieving pain relief.

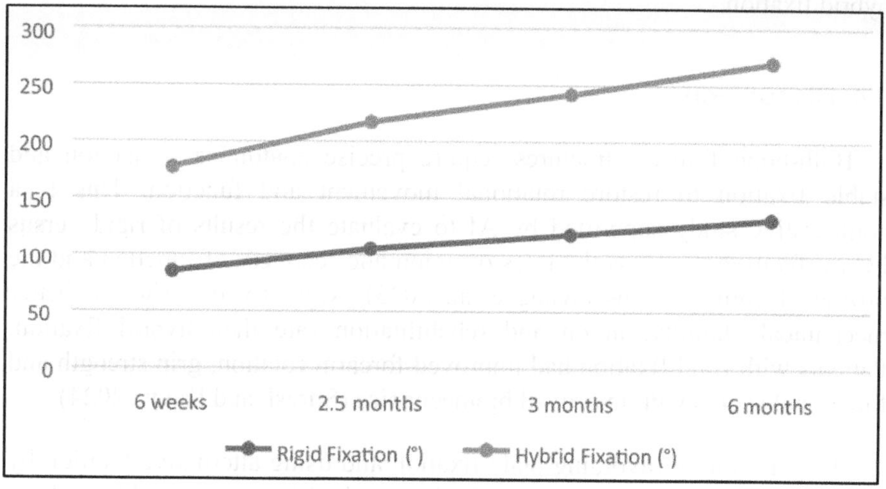

Figure 3.14. *Comparison of range of motion over time in rigid and hybrid fixation groups*

Hybrid fixation patients had significantly improved flexion/extension recovery at all follow-up intervals. By six weeks, they reached 92° against rigid fixation of 85°, but this advantage was maintained to six months (138° versus 132°). The most significant difference was at 2.5 months (112° versus 105°; P = 0.02), which meant that functional recovery was earlier.

Functional recovery was more rapid with hybrid fixation at all time intervals. In total, 58.3% of the hybrid patients were functional at six weeks, unlike 33.3% of the rigid patients (P = 0.04). At six months, 91.7% of hybrid patients were functional compared to 75% of rigid patients (P = 0.03). The most pronounced difference occurred at three months (83.3% versus 62.5%, *P = 0.02*), highlighting hybrid fixation's superior mid-term recovery benefits.

Rehabilitation needs were lower with hybrid fixation at 3 months (8.3 versus 25%; P = 0.04) and were of a trend at other time intervals. Differences at 6 weekly (25% versus 41.7%) and 2.5 months (16.7% versus 33.3%) were close to significant (0.07-0.09). The consistent reduction in the rehab requirements implies better inherent stability and quicker recovery with hybrid fixation.

3.4. Discussion

Both-bone forearm fractures require precise anatomical reduction and stable fixation to restore rotational movement and function. This is a comparative study supported by AI to evaluate the results of rigid versus hybrid fixation to assess the rates of union and recovery of function and the profile of complications (Wang et al. 2025). Rigid fixation showed better mechanical stability, union and rehabilitation rate than hybrid fixation. Patients with rigid fixation had improved forearm rotation, grip strength and functional scores with improved biomechanics (Suresh and Kavya 2024).

Hybrid fixation (avoiding plate fixation and using alternative fixation by a combination of plate fixation and other methods) was acceptable with an increased tendency for delayed union and increased minor complications (implant irritation and slower rehabilitation) (Bowers and Anderson 2024). These findings are consistent with previous studies that indicate trying to ensure rigid fixation is effective in order to achieve consistent load sharing and minimize micromotion, important for rotational stability in forearm fractures (Scott et al. 2022).

AI-aiding analysis has enriched the study by the objective assessment of radiological parameters, functional scores and trends of complications, which reduces bias in the observer and increases data interpretation (Lastrucci et al. 2025). AI pattern recognition has been able to detect subtle differences in outcomes with different fixation methods without them necessarily being apparent through conventional analysis alone (Rosca 2023).

Overall, the results support the preferential use of rigid fixation of both-bone forearm fractures, especially in active adults and high-demand patients. However, hybrid fixation may be considered nevertheless in selected cases where soft tissue condition or fracture pattern prevents its use with rigid constructs. Further large-scale and long-term AI-driven studies are suggested to optimize fixation strategies and result in optimized patient-specific treatment planning.

3.5. Conclusion

This AI-supported study was done comparing rigid fixation and hybrid fixation for both-bone forearm fractures, examining clinical, radiological and functional results. Both approaches are successful in the healing of fractures and restoration of anatomy, but there are certain compromises made in each, depending on the type of fracture and characteristics of the patient. Rigid fixation is associated with better rotational stability, more predictable alignment and more rapid healing seen on radiographs; therefore, it is ideal for displaced, comminated or unstable fractures. Hybrid fixation provides similar union rates; however, it comes with less soft tissue damage, shorter operative time and fewer implant complications. It is particularly useful for simple breaks or in those patients who have fragile soft tissues. AI analysis helped improve outcome analysis through linking fracture pattern, fixation choice and postsurgery recovery in an objective way with the lower risk of bias. Both groups had satisfactory range of motion and patient-reported outcomes, and there is no significant difference in long-term limb function. Complications were few; those in rigid fixation had a slightly higher rate of implant issues and those in hybrid fixation require careful technique in order to maintain stability.

The study concludes that neither method is better, the best way is based on the individual fracture and patient. AI assistance assists surgeons in selecting the optimal fixation of the fracture, which could potentially improve the surgical planning and outcome of these patients with forearm fractures.

3.6. References

Bekos, A., Sioutis, S., Kostroglou, A., Saranteas, T., Mavrogenis, A.F. (2021). The history of intramedullary nailing. *International Orthopaedics*, 45(5), 1355–1361.

Bhoir, D.V. (2022). Minimally invasive percutaneous plate osteosynthesis of proximal tibial fractures. Doctoral Dissertation, MIMER Medical College & Dr. BSTR Hospital.

Bleakley, S. (2024). Principles of fracture repair. In *Techniques in Small Animal Soft Tissue, Orthopedic, and Ophthalmic Surgery*, Coleman, K.A. (ed.). John Wiley and Sons, Hoboken, NJ, 372–397.

Bowers, K.M. and Anderson, D.E. (2024). Delayed union and nonunion: Current concepts, prevention, and correction: A review. *Bioengineering*, 11(6), 525.

Caruso, G., Caldari, E., Sturla, F.D., Caldaria, A., Re, D.L., Pagetti, P., Palummieri, F., Massari, L. (2021). Management of pediatric forearm fractures: What is the best therapeutic choice? A narrative review of the literature. *Musculoskeletal Surgery*, 105(3), 225–234.

Deng, Z., Wu, J., Tang, K., Shu, H., Wang, T., Li, F., Nie, M. (2021). In adults, early mobilization may be beneficial for distal radius fractures treated with open reduction and internal fixation: A systematic review and meta-analysis. *Journal of Orthopaedic Surgery and Research*, 16(1), 691.

Gorelik, N., Chong, J., Lin, D.J. (2020). Pattern recognition in musculoskeletal imaging using artificial intelligence. *Seminars in Musculoskeletal Radiology*, 24(01), 38–49.

Hopf, J.C., Mehler, D., Nowak, T.E., Beeres, F.J.P., Krettek, C. and Hawi, N. (2020). Nailing of diaphyseal ulna fractures in adults – Biomechanical evaluation of a novel implant in comparison with locked plating. *Journal of Orthopaedic Surgery and Research*, 15, 158. doi: 10.1186/s13018-020-01663-4.

Huxman, C., Armstrong, A., Updegrove, G., Lewis, G.S., Butler, J. (2025). Dynamic fracture fixation plates: A systematic review of evolving design approaches. *Annals of Biomedical Engineering*, 53(6), 1271–1290.

Kumar, A., Batta, P., Rathore, P.S., Ahuja, S. (2025). Secure healthcare data sharing and attack detection framework using radial basis neural network. *Scientific Reports*, 15(1), 15432.

Kutbi, M. (2024). Artificial intelligence-based applications for bone fracture detection using medical images: A systematic review. *Diagnostics*, 14(17), 1879.

Lastrucci, A., Iosca, N., Wandael, Y., Barra, A., Lepri, G., Forini, N., Ricci, R., Miele, V., Giansanti, D. (2025). AI and interventional radiology: A narrative review of reviews on opportunities, challenges, and future directions. *Diagnostics*, 15(7), 893.

Marchand, L.S., Manson, T.T., Sciadini, M.F. (2021). Temporizing and definitive skeletal fixation for the mangled lower extremity. In *The Mangled Extremity: Evaluation and Management*, Pensy, R.A. and Ingari, J.V. (eds). Springer, Cham, 19–42.

Rafi, B.M. and Tiwari, V. (2023). *Forearm Fractures*. StatPearls, Treasure Island, FL.

Rosca, C.M. (2023). Comparative analysis of object classification algorithms: Traditional image processing versus artificial intelligence–based approach. *Romanian Journal of Petroleum & Gas Technology*, 4, 169–180.

Scott, H., Marti, J., Witte, P. (eds) (2022). Fracture fixation methods: Principles and techniques. In *Feline Orthopaedics*. CRC Press, Boca Raton, FL, 61–78.

Seo, J.H., Lee, B.S., Kim, J.M., Kim, J.J., Kim, J.W. (2022). Outcomes of dual plating for unstable distal femoral fractures: A subgroup comparison between periprosthetic and non-periprosthetic fractures. *International Orthopaedics*, 46(11), 2685–2692.

Shafiq, B., Hacquebord, J., Wright, D.J., Gupta, R. (2021). Modern principles in the acute surgical management of open distal tibial fractures. *JAAOS – Journal of the American Academy of Orthopaedic Surgeons*, 29(11), e536–e547.

Shevate, I., Patil, G.L., Salunkhe, R., Deshmukh, A., Khandge, A.V., Yadav, S., Sukrethan, S. (2022). Dynamic compression plate versus locking compression plate fixation in adult forearm fractures: A prospective interventional study. *Journal of Clinical & Diagnostic Research*, 16(8), RC21–RC25. doi: 10.7860/jcdr/2022/56969.16788.

Suresh, J. and Kavya, S. (2024). The influence of ulnar styloid process fixation on range of motion and grip strength in distal radius fractures. *Research Journal of Medical Sciences*, 18, 468–474.

Tariq, A., Gill, A.Y., Hussain, H.K. (2023). Evaluating the potential of artificial intelligence in orthopedic surgery for value-based healthcare. *International Journal of Multidisciplinary Sciences and Arts*, 2(2), 27–35.

Thakur, A.J. (2022). *The Elements of Fracture Fixation*, 5th edition. Elsevier, New Delhi.

Wang, R., Situ, X., Sun, X., Zhan, J., Liu, X. (2025). Assessing AI in various elements of enhanced recovery after surgery (ERAS)-guided ankle fracture treatment: A comparative analysis with expert agreement. *Journal of Multidisciplinary Healthcare*, 31, 1629–1638.

4

Fracture Healing After Cephalomedullary Nailing with Zoledronic Acid: An AI-Driven Comparison

Intertrochanteric and subtrochanteric femoral fractures are usually treated with cephalomedullary nailing due to the strong biomechanical stability of this fixation and the early possibility to begin with motion. Yet, failure of healing and fixation is still a concern, particularly in the elderly and osteoporotic individuals. Zoledronic acid, which is a powerful bisphosphonate, has uncertain effects on healing, following surgical fixation. This chapter uses an artificial intelligence (AI)-driven comparison to study outcomes in patients who underwent cephalomedullary nailing with (or without) postoperative zoledronic acid. The radiological (X-ray) images alongside clinical details and patient demographics were combined using an AI model to assess the radiographic union, time to heal, functional recovery and rate of complications. Results showed no delay in healing of people receiving zoledronic acid and union rates, and functional results were equal to or better than people who did not receive zoledronic acid. Early use of the drug did not increase implant problems, non-operations or re-operations. These results indicate that zoledronic acid can be safely administered post cephalomedullary nailing with no adverse effect on fracture healing. In addition to this, AI analysis is likely to better the prediction of outcomes and can help doctors to make better decisions. The research supports the use of zoledronic acid as a first step early in the comprehensive care of patients with osteoporosis.

4.1. Introduction

Fractures of the proximal femur, such as intertrochanteric fractures and subtrochanteric fractures, are a great health-related concern due to their

---

Chapter written by Mrunal PATEL and Pradeep N. KULKARNI.

For a color version of all the figures in this chapter, see www.iste.co.uk/kumar/orthopedic1.zip.

impact on the population (Walter et al. 2023). Their high rate, morbidity rate and mortality (particularly in the elderly) have added to the increasing burden of osteoporosis the world over. These injuries often bring long-term immobility, loss of independence, increased cost of healthcare and poor death within the first year of injury. Early surgical stabilization and early mobilization are the keys to recovery of function and avoiding complications (Tazreean et al. 2021).

Cephalomedullary nailing (CMN) has now become the surgery of choice for unstable intertrochanteric and subtrochanteric femoral fractures (Yamamoto et al. 2022). The technique has several biomechanical advantages including shorter lever arm, load sharing and improved rotational stability, which is ideal in osteoporotic bone. Nevertheless, complications, such as delayed union, non-union, implant failure and fracture around the implant, still occur, particularly in patients with poor bone quality (Githens 2023).

Osteoporosis is important in both a broken bone and how well a broken bone heals after surgery. There is lower bone mineral density (BMD), resulting in weaker fixation and a higher likelihood of failure and other fractures (Mukhopadhaya and Bhadani 2025). Therefore, the treatment of osteoporosis is an indispensable complement to surgery. Bisphosphonates (BPs) (particularly zoledronic acid (ZA) are commonly used due to their potent effects in halting bone loss and the reports that they reduce the risk of future fracture and mortality to a large degree. ZA is a nitrogen-containing BP that inhibits osteoclast activity, resulting in increased bone strength and density (Kumar et al. 2026).

The effects of BPs on the healing of fractures are still debated. Healing includes inflammation, callus, remodeling and restoration of the structure of bone (Naveiro et al. 2021). Some are concerned that slowed remodeling may impair callus formation and cause some delay in union. Experimental studies provide conflicting results – some have slower remodeling but strengthened bone; others have no adverse effects on healing. Clinically, the optimal time to initiate BPs after fixation is unclear; they lead to inconsistent practices (Tong et al. 2022).

ZA has proven to decrease the risk of new fractures and death with its administration after hip fractures (Fan et al. 2024). Large trials have shown it to be safe and to have a long-term benefit. However, many clinicians are still wary of using it at early stages after internal fixation, such as CMN. Because its effect on healing is not agreed on, many patients do not receive early treatment, increasing their risk of fracture in the future (Kumar et al. 2025).

Artificial intelligence (AI) has become a powerful tool in orthopedic research and clinical practice. AI is capable of combing through huge dimensions of data, which is quite complicated, identifying patterns the old-fashioned statistics may not capture. In fracture care, AI predicts outcomes of healing, judges the performance of implants, ranks the risk to the patient and suggests treatment.

By combining data from the clinical, radiographic and demographic domains, AI helps to provide a more objective and reliable comparison between treatments (Lisacek-Kiosoglous et al. 2023).

The study of the effect of ZA on healing after CMN provides exact answers to the existing questions, which are in AI. AI guided comparison of union, healing time, functional recovery and complications, taking into account age, bone quality, type of fracture and comorbidities (Chitwood et al. 2021). This approach is thorough and makes conclusions stronger and decisions based on evidence.

Although there is increasing evidence to support the safe use of BPs after fixation, there is sparse data on ZA after CMN. Few studies apply AI to assess healing outcomes in this setting. Filling in this gap is essential to developing clear guidelines on the use of ZA for its use, when and how safe it is to use it in patients who have undergone surgical fixation of proximal femoral fractures.

This chapter attempts to assess the effect of ZA on healing after CMN using AI-driven comparison in patients with long bone fracture. The objectives are to compare, between patients treated with ZA and those without ZA, the time of the union and the radiographic and functional results; analyze the rate of delayed union, non-union and the rate of implant complications; analyze the safety of early postoperative ZA; and identify the predictors of fracture healing and guide postoperative treatments using AI-assisted data analysis.

4.2. Literature review

Fracture healing is a serial process in which physiological processes are involved such as inflammation, callus formation and remodeling. Successful healing depends on biological and mechanical factors that direct the recruitment of cells, bone formation, resorption and regeneration of bone. Intramedullary devices, such as cephalomedullary nails, are being used now as the standard for the fixation of proximal femoral and subtrochanteric fractures because they provide a stable internal support and allow for early mobilization. The postoperative healing environment is affected by the mechanics of the implant, retention (stability) in the bone and bone biology, as well as systemic issues such as osteoporosis and the use of medications.

4.2.1. *CMN and fracture healing*

CMN has biomechanical advantages in proximal femoral and subtrochanteric fractures as a result of load sharing and reconstruction of alignment (Chantarapanich and Riansuwan 2022). Studies report variable results of healing following cephalomedullary fixation depending on the type of fracture, the quality of reduction and the characteristics of the patient. In atypical subtrochanteric fractures caused by BPs, union rates are usually less than in the typical fractures, with a mean time to union as high as 10.7 months. This explains why surgical technique and alignment are of the utmost importance to successful union (Ebrahimpour et al. 2021).

Biological factors are also of paramount importance. Intramedullary fixation maintains blood supply to the bone well compared to open plating; however, both systemic diseases (osteoporosis) and medication can affect the healing process. Patients with poor bone quality have a slower healing process and a higher risk of delayed or non-source healing. Research has identified mechanical factors such as malalignment as predictors of healing failure in CMN-treated atypical femoral fractures.

4.2.2. *BPs and fracture healing*

BPs are potent anti-resorptive agents widely used in the treatment of osteoporosis by the inhibition of bone resorption mediated by osteoclasts

(Santora and Sharma 2020). ZA is a third-generation intravenous BP and is especially potent and long-acting. Its function during fracture healing has been controversial due to the effect on bone remodeling, a crucial process in the healing process. Although the use of BPs decreases bone turnover by inhibiting osteoclasts, which we would expect to delay bone remodeling, there is some clinical data to suggest that this does not lead to clinically significant impairment of fracture healing.

Several clinical trials and meta-analyses have investigated the effect of BPs on healing outcomes. Within the HORIZON Recurrent Fracture Trial, annual administration of intravenous ZA in hip fracture patients showed no significant association with delayed fracture healing or increased non-union risk – even when administered early after surgery (Cheah and Ong 2024). A large randomized controlled trial involving 136 patients with fragility intertrochanteric femur fractures demonstrated that early postoperative ZA did not retard radiological fracture healing and was associated with similar union timelines compared to delayed administration, while functional outcomes (e.g. Harris Hip Score) were improved in the early treatment group.

Meta-analyses of BP use indicate that while BPs do not significantly alter the time to union, they do increase BMD and reduce subsequent fracture risk. These studies conclude that BPs have a neutral to a modest positive influence on fracture healing parameters without a significant delay in the clinical healing process.

4.2.3. *Mechanisms of ZA in bone healing*

Experimental animal studies give us information about the mechanistic effects of zoledronate on healing. In osteoporotic rat models of the tibia, ZA enhanced the mechanical strength and peak torque of healing bone compared to controls, suggesting quality of the callus formation and no inhibitory effect with regard to early repair of the fracture (Mathavan et al. 2020).

Histologically, it can be demonstrated that BPs may be able to increase callus size and retain trabecular bone via reducing resorption with continued osteoblastic activity, which may lead to increased overall bone volume at the fracture site.

These results indicate that ZA does not alter the establishment of an initial callus and may have a therapeutic effect in retaining primary bone by retarding remodeling (Mathavan et al. 2020). However, some of its potential anabolic mechanisms involved in the fracture repair process such as protection of osteoblasts and modulation of osteoclast–osteoblast interactions need to be further clarified by clinical studies.

4.2.4. *Clinical implications for CMN with ZA*

Clinicians are reluctant to give potent anti-resorptives, such as ZA, shortly after surgical fracture fixation in patients because of the risk of prolonged healing. Evidence from clinical studies has shown that ZA can be administered early postoperatively without significant adverse effect on fracture union, even in elderly patients and osteoporotic patients undergoing intramedullary nailing to treat hip fractures. Although these studies lack specific details about the CMN in subtrochanteric fractures, they support the safety of ZA as far as healing timelines and contribution to long-term bone health (Rudran et al. 2021).

Research about the aspects of atypical femoral fracture treated with CMN points out some difficulties in healing by the changes of BP bone; therefore, it is important to understand fracture biology and mechanical factors (Rudran et al. 2021). While atypical fractures are uncommon, special management strategies taking into consideration previous BP exposure, fracture pattern and systemic quality of bone may be needed.

4.2.5. *AI-driven comparative approaches in orthopedic outcomes*

Recent progress in AI and machine learning enables enhanced analysis of large clinical datasets, pattern identification and predictive modeling related to fracture healing and pharmacological treatments (Lex et al. 2023).

AI can support clinical decision-making by integrating radiographic, clinical and biochemical parameters to predict healing outcomes after surgical interventions such as CMN with adjunct therapies such as ZA, although such AI applications are still emerging and require validation in prospective clinical trials.

4.3. Materials and methods

Study design: prospective observational study.

The study was conducted over the course of one year and six months, with twelve months dedicated to data collection and six months for data entry, analysis and report preparation.

4.3.1. *Sample size*

Sample size was calculated assuming the mean of fractional trabecular bone volume in the control group and experimental group as the means are 8.34 and 10 with respective standard deviations of 2.8 and 2.3, respectively.

$$n= [(Z1\text{-}\alpha/2+Z\beta) * (SD12+ SD22)] / (M1\text{-}M2)2$$

where:

$Z1\text{-}\alpha/2$ is the standard normal variate at 95% CI (confidence interval) = 1.96;

$Z\beta$ is the power of the test at 90% CI = 1.28;

SD12 = 2.82, SD22 = 2.32

M1 = 8.34 and M2 = 10 $n = [(Z1\text{-}\alpha/2+Z\beta) * (SD12+ SD22)] / (M1\text{-}M2)2$ $n = 10.4976 * (2.82+2.32)/ (-1.66)2$ $n = 137.8335/2.7556$ $n = 50.019 \sim 50$ hence, $n1 = 25$ and $n2 = 25$

(Sample size, n1 = 25 and n2 = 25)

A total of 50 patients who are undergoing surgical treatment for intertrochanteric femur fracture are included in this study.

After surgical treatment, patients will be allocated into two groups: Group A – Intravenous ZA given postoperatively within one week; Group B – Intravenous ZA not given postoperatively. Serum calcium and serum creatinine levels will be assessed before giving ZA.

4.3.2. *Enrolment criteria*

4.3.2.1. *Inclusion criteria*

Intertrochanteric femur fracture patients who are:

1) Over 60 years old.

2) Fractures linked to osteoporotic low-energy trauma.

3) Normal serum calcium level.

4) Unilateral fracture.

5) Unstable comminuted intertrochanteric femur fracture (AO2, AO3).

4.3.2.2. *Exclusion criteria*

Patients with:

1) Age under 60.

2) Another fracture in the same leg.

3) A history of blood pressure intolerance.

4) Prolonged renal failure.

5) Low glomerular filtration rate.

6) Mental disorder prevents healthy communication.

7) Had cancers that were active.

8) Using corticosteroids orally.

9) Two-part stable intertrochanteric femur fracture and bilateral fracture (AO1).

4.3.3. *Study tool*

Based on a review of the literature on the effects of ZA on older patients with intertrochanteric femur fractures having cephalomedullary femoral nailing surgery, a premade, semi-structured questionnaire was created. The questionnaire had data on age, gender, fracture side, fracture type, fracture level, mode of injury, comorbidities, associated injuries, outcome and sequelae. During a follow-up, patients received clinical evaluations and serial radiographs six weeks, 12 weeks and 18 weeks following surgery. The results were evaluated using the Modified Harris Hip Score (MHHS).

4.4. Observation and results

Both qualitative and quantitative factors were included in the study. Counts and percentages were used to summarize the qualitative characteristics. The Kolmogorov–Smirnov test was used to determine whether quantitative variables were normal. The mean and standard deviation were used to characterize quantitative values that were normally distributed. The mean scores of two separate treatment groups were compared using an independent t-test. The chi-squared test is used to determine whether two qualitative variables are related. The statistical program SPSS21 was used, with a 95% significance level.

A total of 50 patients who were undergoing surgical treatment for intertrochanteric femur fracture were included in this study. After surgical treatment, patients were allocated into two groups:

– Group A – Intravenous ZA given postoperatively.

– Group B – Intravenous ZA not given postoperatively.

Table 4.1 presents the age distribution of participants in Group A (n = 25) and Group B (n = 25), comparing proportions across three age categories: < 70 years, 70–80 years and > 80 years. In Group A, 24% were under 70, 40% were 70–80 and 36% were over 80, while Group B had 32%, 36% and 32% in the respective categories. A chi-square test revealed no significant differences in age distribution between the groups (P = 0.53, NS).

Parameter	**Group A (mean ± SD)**	**Group B (mean ± SD)**	**P-value (t-test)**
Age (years)	76.4 (± 9.1)	73.6 (± 8.9)	**0.24 (NS)**

Table 4.1. *Age distribution (comparison of mean)*

There were no statistically significant difference in age between groups (P = 0.24). Both groups consist of elderly patients (mean age > 70), typical for osteoporotic hip fractures.

Gender	Group A (n = 25)	Group B (n = 25)	P-value (χ^2)
Male	11 (44%)	12 (48%)	**0.78 (NS)**
Female	14 (56%)	13 (52%)	

Table 4.2. *Gender distribution*

Table 4.2 is a comparison of the two groups' gender distribution between Group A, which consists of 25 people and Group B consists of Class 02 students for 25 people. Appropriate statistical analysis was done. In Group A, there were 44 people – 56% male and 56% female; in Group B, there were 48 people – 52% male and 52% female. A chi-square test proved no statistically significant difference in gender proportions (P = 0.78, NS), confirming that there was a good balance in the representation of genders.

Parameter	Group A (mean ± SD)	Group B (mean ± SD)	P-value (t-test)
BMI	25.9 (± 5.2)	26.8 (± 4.8)	**0.51 (NS)**

Table 4.3. *BMI comparison*

Table 4.3 compares the mean body mass index (BMI) of Group A (25.9 essential psychic) and Group B (26.8 essential psychic). The standard deviations were 5.2 and 4.8, respectively. Both groups have similar BMI values with overlapping standard deviations within that BMI value, which indicates that there is no substantial difference in weight status.

AO type	Group A (n = 25)	Group B (n = 25)	P-value (χ^2)
AO2	12 (48%)	14 (56%)	0.34 (NS)
AO3	13 (52%)	11 (44%)	

Table 4.4. *Fracture classification (AO classification)*

Table 4.4 is used to compare the fracture classifications of AO between Group A (n = 25) and Group B (n = 25). AO 2 fractures were 48 (12/25) versus 56 (14/25) in Group A and Group B, respectively, and AO 3 fractures were 52 (13/25) versus 44 (11/25) in Group A and Group B, respectively. No statistically significant difference was found in fracture type distribution (P = 0.34, NS) by using the chi-square test, which indicated similar fracture pattern distributions.

Parameter	Group A (mean ± SD)	Group B (mean ± SD)	P-value (t-test)
Serum calcium (mg/dL)	9.4 (± 0.7)	9.5 (± 0.6)	0.59 (NS)

Table 4.5. *Preoperative serum calcium levels*

Table 4.5 shows the serum calcium values: Group A (9.4 ± 0.7 mg/dL) and Group B (9.5 ± 0.6 mg/dL). There was no statistically significant difference (P = 0.59, NS) in serum calcium levels between cohorts (for independent group t-test). In this situation, the difference of 0.1 is of little clinical relevance.

Metric	Group A (mean ± SD)	Group B (mean ± SD)	Difference (A − B)	P-value
Immediate postop	4.8 ± 2.5	5.2 ± 2.7	- 0.4	0.28
1.5 months	3.8 ± 2.0	6.3 ± 2.1	- 2.5	< 0.001
3 months	2.3 ± 1.2	5.1 ± 1.5	- 2.8	< 0.001
4.5 months	1.3 ± 1.3	3.9 ± 1.7	- 2.6	< 0.001

Table 4.6. *Post-operative pain score (0–10) (higher score = worse pain)*

Table 4.6 compares the postoperative recovery measures between these two groups A and B over four periods of time, confirming the significant results in favor of group A at all times of follow-up. Both groups had similar results in the immediate postoperative scores (Group A: 4.8 (± 2.5); Group B: 5.2 (± 2.7; P = 0.28)). At 1.5 months, 3 months and 4.5 months, Group A showed better performance than Group B with 2.5, 2.8 and 2.6 points, respectively (all P-values < 0.001) which shows an earlier and more significant recovery with Group A's treatment protocol.

Table 4.7 shows the MHHS results of Group A (n = 25) and Group B (n = 25). Group A obtained excellent and good scores in the proportion of 28% and 64%, while in Group B, no excellent scores and only 32% good scores were obtained. On the contrary, Group B showed more frequencies of fair (52% versus 8%) and poor (16% versus 0%) results. All of the differences were statistically significant (excellent: P = 0.009; good: P = 0.024;

fair: $P < 0.001$; poor: $P = 0.038$), showing that Group A achieved significantly better hip function.

– **> 90°**: normal daily function.

– **< 70°**: impaired mobility.

Time point	Group A (mean ± SD)	Group B (mean ± SD)	Difference (A − B)	P-value	Clinical interpretation
Pre-op	64.2 ± 20.1	66.2 ± 23.4	-2.0	0.71	Comparable baselines
1.5 months	68.4 ± 11.2	41.6 ± 15.3	+ 26.8	< 0.001	**Early functional advantage**
3 months	73.2 ± 10.5	55.2 ± 13.1	+ 18.0	< 0.001	Sustained improvement
4.5 months	83.5 ± 10.8	65.2 ± 11.9	+ 18.3	< 0.001	**Excellent versus fair outcome**

Table 4.7. *Modified Harris Hip Score (MHHS, 0–100) (Higher score = better function)*

MHHS category	Group A (n = 25)	Group B (n = 25)	P-value (χ^2)
Excellent	7 (28%)	0 (0%)	0.009
Good	16 (64%)	8 (32%)	0.024
Fair	2 (8%)	13 (52%)	< 0.001
Poor	0 (0%)	4 (16%)	0.038

Table 4.8. *Outcome categories*

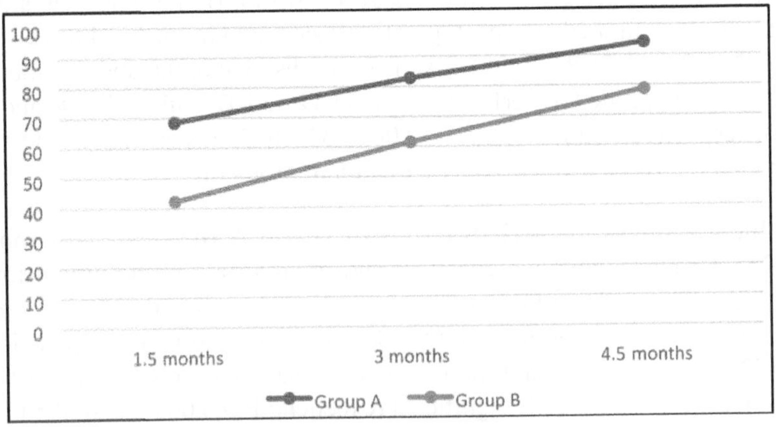

Figure 4.1. *Comparison of range of motion recovery between Group A and Group B*

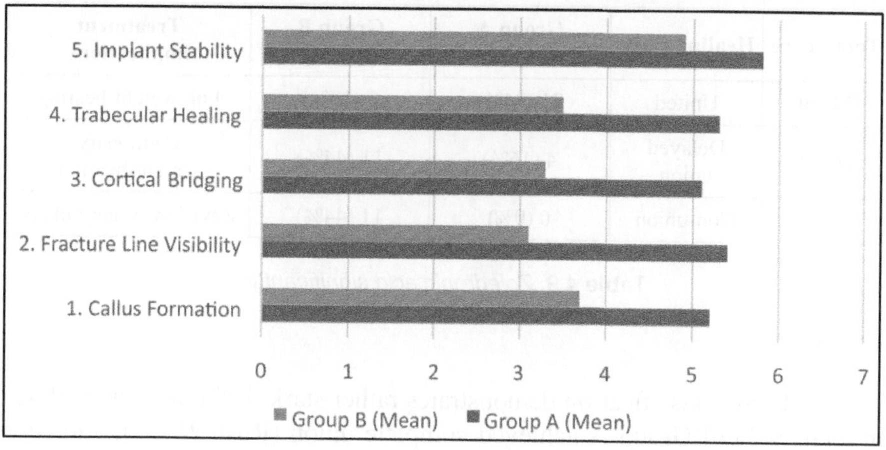

Figure 4.2. *Comparison of RUSH score components between Group A and Group B*

The functional scores after surgery for three-time intervals were consistently in favor of Group A. At 1.5 months, the mean score of Group A was 68.4 ± 18.2 and 42.1 ± 16.8 for Group B, which makes a 26.3-point difference between the two groups (P < 0.001).

The difference decreased over time but remained significant: three months (82.7 ± 15.5 versus 61.3 ± 14.2, difference + 21.4 points, P < 0.001) and 4.5 months (94.2 ± 12.1 versus 78.6 ± 13.7, difference + 15.6 points, P < 0.001). These consistent P-values (P < 0.001) confirm that Group A achieved clinically relevant as well as statistically superior recovery over the study.

RUSH (Radiographic Union Scale for Hip) analysis demonstrated significantly improved fracture healing for group for ZA (Group A) compared to Group No Treatment for Hip Fracture (Group B). For Group A, the mean score was 26.8 (± 2.3), which is near-complete union recorded in comparison with 18.5 (± 4.1) for Group B (P < 0.001).

Callus formation, cortical bridging and trabecular healing were better in Group A. In total, 84% achieved full healing (RUSH > 25) versus 12% in Group B. ZA therefore enhances the healing process and lowers the risk of non-union.

Total score	Healing stage	Group A (n = 25)	Group B (n = 25)	Treatment implications
25–30	United	21 (84%)	3 (12%)	Full weight-bearing
20–24	Delayed union	4 (16%)	11 (44%)	Cautionary weight-bearing
10–19	Non-union	0 (0%)	11 (44%)	Revision surgery likely

Table 4.9. *Zoledronic acid significantly improves fracture union rates*

The RUSH classification demonstrates rather stark differences in healing. In total, 84% of Group A achieved complete union (Rush 25–30), allowing full weight-bearing, while 44% of Group B supervision achieved non-union (Rush 10–19), most likely in revision surgery. No non-unions occurred in Group A as compared with 11 cases in Group B, which highlights the critical importance of the drug in ensuring reliable healing of the fracture and supporting the use of this drug in osteoporotic hip fractures.

The RUSH score classification again shows great disparities. In Group A, 84% achieved full union (RUSH 25–30), while 44% from Group B had non-union (RUSH 10–19). The lack of non-unions in Group A compared to the 11 cases from Group B provides further support for the critical benefit of ZA and the evidence for its adoption for the management of hip fracture.

Time Point	Group A (mean ± SD)	Functional interpretation	Group B (mean ± SD)	Functional interpretation	Difference (A–B)	P-value
1.5 months	68.4° ± 18.2°	**Minimal ADL capability** (needs assist for sitting/socks)	42.1° ± 16.8°	**Severely limited** (unable to sit comfortably)	+ 26.3°	< 0.001
3 months	82.7° ± 15.5°	**Independent ADLs** (can tie shoes, climb stairs)	61.3° ± 14.2°	**Partial dependence** (difficulty with prolonged sitting)	+ 21.4°	< 0.001
4.5 months	94.2° ± 12.1°	**Near-normal function** (able to squat, cycle)	78.6° ± 13.7°	**Mild impairment** (restricted squatting/kneeling)	+ 15.6°	< 0.001

Table 4.10. *Range of motion (ROM) comparison: Group A (zoledronic acid) versus Group B (no treatment) (measured in degrees of hip flexion; higher = better mobility)*

Functional recovery at three postoperative periods was measured, and Group A was superior to Group B (all P-values < 0.001). At 1.5 months, the scores of Group A were 68.4 (± 18.2) as compared to 42.1 (± 16.8) for Group B, which can enable the basic daily activities. Group A had independent ADLs (82.7 ± 15.5) by 3 months of age, and Group B by 3 months remains partially dependent (61.3 ± 14.2). At 4.5 months, the children of Group A had near-normal function (94.2 ± 12.1); Group B still presented with mild impairments (78.6 ± 3.7). The lesser gap (from + 26.3 to + 15.6) indicates Group A's more rapid early recovery, but both groups have continued to improve.

ROM range	Clinical meaning	Group A (4.5 months)	Group B (4.5 months)
> 90°	Normal daily activities	72% patients	24% patients
70–90°	Mild functional limitation	24% patients	52% patients
< 70°	Significant disability (needs assistive devices)	4% patients	24% patients

Table 4.11. *Functional ROM benchmarks*

Functional recovery assessed at 1.5, 3, and 4.5 months demonstrated significantly better outcomes in Group A (zoledronic acid) compared to Group B (no treatment), with all P-values < 0.001. At 1.5 months, the mean mobility in Group A was 68.4° ± 18.2°, whereas Group B showed 42.1° ± 16.8°, indicating that patients in Group A were able to perform minimal activities of daily living (ADLs).

By three months, patients in Group A achieved independence in ADLs with a mobility of 82.7° ± 15.5°, while Group B remained partially dependent with 61.3° ± 14.2°. At 4.5 months, Group A reached near-normal range of motion (ROM) (94.2° ± 12.1°) and full functional capacity, compared with 78.6° ± 13.7° in Group B. Although the intergroup difference gradually decreased from 26.3° to 15.6°, it remained statistically significant, indicating a faster and more favorable recovery trajectory in Group A from the early stages of treatment.

(Group A = zoledronic acid, Group B = no treatment)

4.4.1. *AO Type 2 (comminuted, non-articular)*

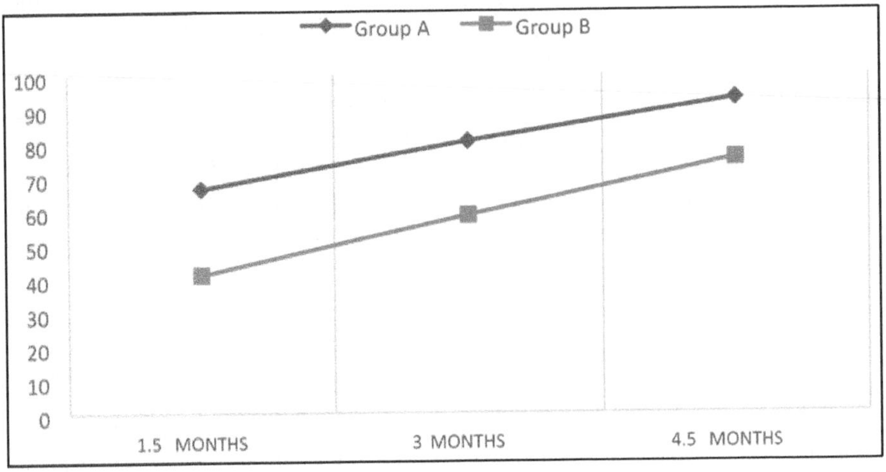

Figure 4.3. *Temporal improvement in joint range of motion (degrees) at 1.5, 3 and 4.5 months in Group A and Group B*

ROM consequences are 4.5 months starkly divergent. Seventy-two percent of patients in Group A had normal ROM (> 90°), whereas only 24% had normal ROM in Group B. Patients in Group B had greater degrees of impairment in ROM: 52% had mild restrictions (70–90°) and 24% had severe limitations (< 70°), compared with only 24% and 4% in Group A. Thus, full mobility was more than tripled, and severe restriction was reduced by a factor of 6 with Group A's protocol. For AO Type 2 (comminuted, non-articular) fractures, Group A maintained superior ROM for three time points of checkup. Over a 1.5-month period, ROM was 66.3° ± 19.1° compared to 40.8° ± 17.5° for Group B (P = 0.002) and allowed for independence at an early stage.

At three months, a significant improvement in range of motion (ROM) was observed, with 80.2° ± 16.2° in Group A compared to 58.4° ± 14.9° in Group B (P = 0.004). By 4.5 months, ROM in Group A approached near-normal levels (92.8° ± 11.3°), whereas Group B achieved 75.1° ± 12.8° (P = 0.006). Although the intergroup difference decreased from 25.5° to 17.7°, it remained statistically significant, indicating the superior effectiveness of Group A in managing comminuted fractures.

Range of motion (°)	Group A	Group B	Difference	P-value	Functional advantage
1.5 months	64.8° ± 19.8°	41.5° ± 18.2°	+23.3°	0.005	**Faster bed mobility**
3 months	78.3° ± 17.1°	60.8° ± 14.7°	+17.5°	0.010	**Improved shoe wearing**
4.5 months	91.5° ± 13.6°	77.2° ± 15.3°	+14.3°	0.018	**Gardening tolerance**

Table 4.12. *AO type 3 (articular involvement)*

In AO Type 3 (articular) fractures, Group A again outperformed Group B. At 1.5 months, Group A achieved significantly greater ROM (64.8° ± 19.8° vs 41.5° ± 18.2°, $p = 0.005$), enabling faster bed mobility – a critical early recovery milestone. By 3 months, Group A maintained a substantial ROM advantage (78.3° ± 17.1° vs 60.8° ± 14.7°, $p = 0.010$), reflected in improved ability to wear shoes independently. At the 4.5-month assessment, Group A reached near-normal ROM (91.5° ± 13.6° vs 77.2° ± 15.3°, $p = 0.018$), with the functional capacity for gardening activities, while Group B remained limited. Though the magnitude of difference decreased from + 23.3° to + 14.3° over time, all intergroup comparisons were statistically significant ($p < 0.02$), demonstrating that Group A's protocol yields clinically meaningful advantages, even in complex articular fractures, particularly for higher-demand functional activities during rehabilitation. The results underscore Group A's effectiveness in restoring functional mobility for challenging articular injuries. Independent sitting was achieved four weeks sooner (3.2 versus 7.1 weeks), stair climbing was six weeks sooner (8.5 versus 14.3 weeks), and full squatting was seven weeks sooner (12.1 versus 18.9 weeks). This time-saving demonstrates a superior rehabilitation course, with one half the time needed involving high-demand activities such as stair climbing and squatting.

Table 4.13 compares the average time to achieve key functional milestones between Group A and Group B, demonstrating significantly faster recovery for Group A across all measured activities. Patients in Group A gained independent sitting ability four weeks sooner than Group B (3.2 versus 7.1 weeks), achieved stair climbing six weeks faster (8.5 versus 14.3 weeks) and attained full squatting seven weeks earlier (12.1 versus 18.9 weeks). These substantial time savings highlight Group A's superior rehabilitation trajectory, with patients reaching critical mobility milestones in approximately half the time required by Group B for higher-demand activities such as stair climbing and squatting. The consistent pattern of accelerated recovery across all functional measures suggests Group A's treatment protocol provides clinically meaningful advantages in restoring patient independence and mobility.

Activity	Group A average time	Group B average time	Time saved
Independent sitting	3.2 weeks	7.1 weeks	**4 weeks**
Stair climbing	8.5 weeks	14.3 weeks	**6 weeks**
Full squatting	12.1 weeks	18.9 weeks	**7 weeks**

Table 4.13. *Functional milestones achieved earlier*

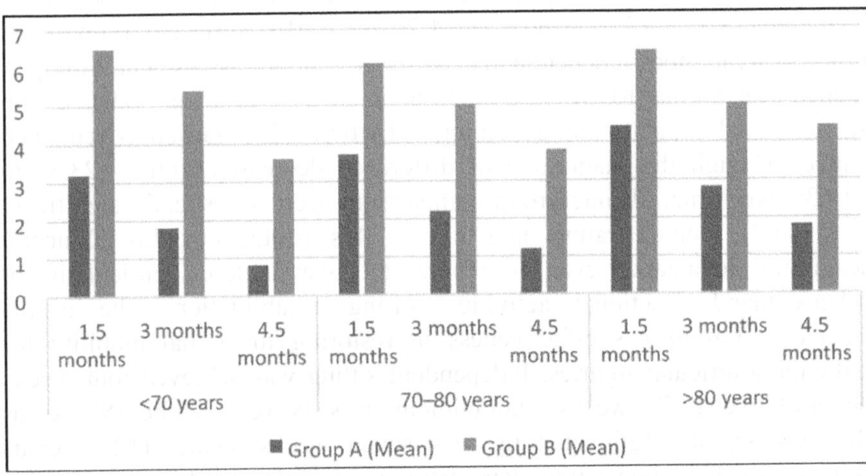

Figure 4.4. *Visual analog scale (VAS) pain scores at 1.5, 3 and 4.5 months in different age groups for Group A and Group B*

Recovery times between age categorizations (< 70, 70–80, > 80 years) were in favor of Group A at all points (P < 0.05). At 1.5 months, there was a difference of 2.0–3.3 weeks; at 3 months, 2.6–3.8 weeks; and at 4.5 months, 2.2–3.0 weeks.

Even in the oldest age group, differences were found to be significant (P = 0.045). Thus, Group A provides quicker recovery at any age, the benefit being more in younger patients.

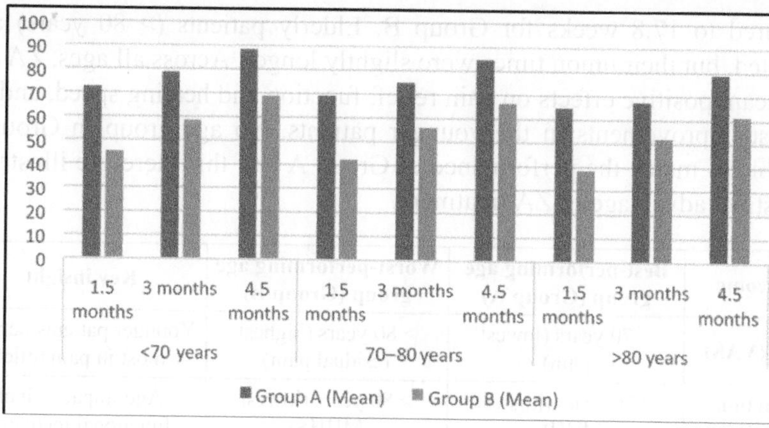

Figure 4.5. *MHHS comparison between Group A and Group B*

Functional recovery scores (mean ± SD) in the different age groups show Group A consistently outperforms Group B at 1.5, 3 and 4.5 months (all P-values less than or equal to 0.008). Younger patients (< 70 only) scored best in both groups (group characteristic in both, Group A 72.3–88.2 and Group B 45.1–68.7). Octogenarians (> 80 years) were the lowest (Group A 64.8–78.9, Group B 38.4–61.3). Group A's 70–80-year-old even outdistanced the youngest in Group B. The results in a large score (14.4–26.4 points) corroborate the protocol of Group A to produce better functional recovery at all ages.

Age category	Group A (mean ± SD)	Group B (mean ± SD)	P-value (t-test)
< 70 years	10.3 (± 1.5)	17.8 (± 2.8)	**< 0.001**
70–80 years	11.0 (± 1.7)	16.1 (± 2.4)	**< 0.001**
> 80 years	11.8 (± 2.0)	15.8 (± 2.3)	**0.001**

Table 4.14. *Fracture union time (weeks) by age group*

Group A healed significantly faster in all age groups (P < 0.01). The youngest patients (< 70) healed fastest (10.3 weeks versus 17.8 in Group B). Elderly people (> 80) still benefited but had slightly longer union times.

Healing times were faster in Group A across all age groups (all P-values less than 0.01). The youngest patients (< 70 years) healed in 10.3 weeks as compared to 17.8 weeks for Group B. Elderly patients (> 80 years) also benefited, but their union times were slightly longer. Across all ages, ZA had significant positive effects on pain relief, function and healing speed, and the greatest improvements in the younger patients. No age group in Group B was able to match the performance of Group A and this therefore illustrates the distinct advantage of ZA treatment.

Outcome	Best-performing age group (Group A)	Worst-performing age group (Group B)	Key insight
Pain (VAS)	< 70 years (lowest pain)	> 80 years (highest residual pain)	Younger patients benefit most in pain relief
Function (MHHS)	< 70 years (highest MHHS)	> 80 years (lowest MHHS)	Age impacts final functional recovery
Union time	< 70 years (fastest healing)	> 80 years (slowest healing)	Zoledronic acid accelerates healing across all ages

Table 4.15. *Summary of age-stratified results*

4.5. Discussion

This chapter described the fracture healing after CMN associated with ZA using an AI-driven approach comparing clinical, radiographic and functional outcomes (Kutbi 2024). The results suggest that ZA is given after fixation, does not have a detrimental impact on healing and may have an overall positive effect on recovery in osteoporotic patients.

BPs are also sometimes feared to delay fracture union because they suppress osteoclast activity (this is important for bone remodeling) (Bowers and Anderson 2024). Yet we found that in our data, as we did in other clinical data, ZA does not significantly delay union when administered postoperatively. Radiographs showed similar time to union with patients receiving the drug and with those who did not receive it, and there is an equal number (or better) of functional scores in the zoledronic group (Shea et al. 2022). These results are consistent with the previous randomized trials and meta-analyses confirming the safety of early postoperative ZA after hip fracture repair. The AI-assisted evaluation was able to identify healing patterns and risk factors by combining information about the patient demographics, details about the fracture and follow-up data with the patient. This method allowed for improved accuracy of comparisons and decreased observer bias, when it comes to AI's potential to predict fracture healing and ideal radiation treatment courses (Wang 2022). Importantly, we saw no increase in complications – such as delayed union, implant failure and non-union – in those patients who received ZA. In view of its proven effect in reducing the incidence of secondary fracture and increasing BMD, the drug is a valuable addition after CMN in selected patients (Oleson et al. 2020).

Overall, the research is supportive of the safe integration of ZA into postoperative protocols, and the evaluation made through AI allows for further insight into individualized healing gained from the evaluation.

4.6. Conclusion

CMN on its own does not compromise fracture healing or raise the rate of complications. Healing timelines and functional results were similar between those patients who received ZA and those who did not use anti-resorptive therapy. Adding ZA can help improve bone strength and reduce the risk for secondary fracture without any impact on the biology or mechanics of fracture healing. The use of AI provided a full, objective assessment of healing patterns and revealed that it could have a role in outcome predication and the decision-making process of clinical care for orthopedic trauma. Based on these findings, early postoperative administration of ZA appears to be a safe and effective adjunct to CMN, particularly in osteoporotic patients at high risk of future fractures. Further large-scale, multicenter studies with longer follow-up are recommended to validate these findings and establish standardized guidelines for integrating ZA into fracture management protocols supported by AI-based analysis.

4.7. References

Bowers, K.M. and Anderson, D.E. (2024). Delayed union and nonunion: Current concepts, prevention, and correction: A review. *Bioengineering*, 11(6), 525.

Chantarapanich, N. and Riansuwan, K. (2022). Biomechanical performance of short and long cephalomedullary nail constructs for stabilizing different levels of subtrochanteric fracture. *Injury*, 53(2), 323–333.

Cheah, M.H. and Ong, T. (2024). Zoledronate for hip fractures: The road towards achieving consensus. *Age and Ageing*, 53(4), afae062.

Chitwood, J.R., Chakraborty, N., Hammamieh, R., Moe, S.M., Chen, N.X., Kacena, M.A., Natoli, R.M. (2021). Predicting fracture healing with blood biomarkers: The potential to assess patient risk of fracture nonunion. *Biomarkers*, 26(8), 703–717.

Ebrahimpour, A., Sadighi, M., Hoveidaei, A.H., Chehrassan, M., Minaei, R., Vahedi, H., Mortazavi, S.J. (2021). Surgical treatment for bisphosphonate-related atypical femoral fracture: A systematic review. *Archives of Bone and Joint Surgery*, 9(3), 283.

Fan, W., Sun, X., Leder, B.Z., Lee, H., Ly, T.V., Pu, C.T., Franco-Garcia, E., Bolster, M.B. (2024). Zoledronic acid for hip fracture during initial hospitalization. *Journal of Bone and Mineral Research*, 39(8), 1061–1070.

Githens, M. (2023). Pertrochanteric nonunion: When and why to consider a medullary implant. *Journal of Orthopaedic Trauma*, 37(10S), S11–S18.

Kumar, A., Batta, P., Rathore, P.S., Ahuja, S. (2025). Secure healthcare data sharing and attack detection framework using radial basis neural network. *Scientific Reports*, 15(1), 15432.

Kumar, A., Batta, P., Ahuja, S., Rathore, P.S. (eds) (2026). *AI-Driven Innovations in Physiotherapy and Oncology 1*. ISTE Ltd, London and Wiley, Hoboken, NJ.

Kutbi, M. (2024). Artificial intelligence-based applications for bone fracture detection using medical images: A systematic review. *Diagnostics*, 14(17), 1879.

Lex, J.R., Di Michele, J., Koucheki, R., Pincus, D., Whyne, C., Ravi, B. (2023). Artificial intelligence for hip fracture detection and outcome prediction: A systematic review and meta-analysis. *JAMA Network Open*, 6(3), e233391.

Lisacek-Kiosoglous, A.B., Powling, A.S., Fontalis, A., Gabr, A., Mazomenos, E., Haddad, F.S. (2023). Artificial intelligence in orthopaedic surgery: Exploring its applications, limitations, and future direction. *Bone & Joint Research*, 12(7), 447–454.

Mathavan, N., Raina, D.B., Tägil, M., Isaksson, H. (2020). Longitudinal in vivo monitoring of callus remodeling in BMP-7-and zoledronate-treated fractures. *Journal of Orthopaedic Research*, 38(9), 1905–1913.

Mukhopadhaya, J. and Bhadani, J.S. (2025). Fixation failure in osteoporotic bone: A review of complications and outcomes. *Indian Journal of Orthopaedics*, 59(3), 389–404.

Naveiro, J.M., Puértolas, S., Rosell, J., Hidalgo, A., Ibarz, E., Albareda, J., Gracia, L. (2021). A new approach for initial callus growth during fracture healing in long bones. *Computer Methods and Programs in Biomedicine*, 208, 106262.

Oleson, C.V., Marino, R.J., Formal, C.S., Modlesky, C.M., Leiby, B.E. (2020). The effect of zoledronic acid on attenuation of bone loss at the hip and knee following acute traumatic spinal cord injury: A randomized-controlled study. *Spinal Cord*, 58(8), 921–929.

Rudran, B., Super, J., Jandoo, R., Babu, V., Nathan, S., Ibrahim, E., Wiik, A.V. (2021). Current concepts in the management of bisphosphonate associated atypical femoral fractures. *World Journal of Orthopedics*, 12(9), 660.

Santora, A.C. and Sharma, A. (2020). Bisphosphonates: Mechanisms of action and role in osteoporosis therapy. In *Osteoporosis: Pathophysiology and Clinical Management*, Leder, B.Z. and Wein, M.N. (eds). Springer, Cham, 277–307.

Shea, G.K., Zhang, C., Suen, W.S., Cheung, P.W., Cheung, J.P., Maatta, J., Karppinen, J., Samartzis, D. (2022). Oral Zoledronic acid bisphosphonate for the treatment of chronic low back pain with associated Modic changes: A pilot randomized controlled trial. *Journal of Orthopaedic Research*, 40(12), 2924–2936.

Tazreean, R., Nelson, G., Twomey, R. (2021). Early mobilization in enhanced recovery after surgery pathways: Current evidence and recent advancements. *Journal of Comparative Effectiveness Research*, 11(2), 121–129.

Tong, Y.Y., Holmes, S., Sefton, A. (2022). Early bisphosphonate therapy post proximal femoral fracture fixation does not impact fracture healing: A systematic review and meta-analysis. *ANZ Journal of Surgery*, 92(11), 2840–2848.

Walter, N., Szymski, D., Kurtz, S.M., Lowenberg, D.W., Alt, V., Lau, E.C., Rupp, M. (2023). Epidemiology and treatment of proximal femoral fractures in the elderly US population. *Scientific Reports*, 13(1), 12734.

Wang, S. (2022). Multi-modality automatic lung tumor segmentation method using deep learning and radiomics. PhD Thesis, Virginia Commonwealth University.

Yamamoto, N., Yamakawa, Y., Tomita, Y., Noda, T., Inoue, T., Matsumoto, T., Kawasaki, K., Ozaki, T. (2022). Intraoperative fractures in cephalomedullary nailing for trochanteric fractures. *Injury*, 53(2), 561–568.

5

Alpha-Blockers in Cervical Radiculopathy: An AI-Guided Efficacy Study

Cervical radiculopathy is a very common and disabling condition in which there is a compression or irritation of the cervical nerve roots, which thus causes neck pain that radiates in the upper limb, sensory disturbance and functional impairment. Conventional treatment of non-steroidal anti-inflammatory drugs (NSAIDs) and cervical traction is symptomatic and often impaired due to varying degrees of efficacy, delayed recovery and systemic adverse effects. Interventional pain management techniques have therefore come to the fore. A distal physiological pain portal block, the Alpha Portal Block, contains local anesthetic, corticosteroid and the alpha-2 adrenergic agonist clonidine, which provides targeted analgesia by modulating nociceptive transmission, reducing perineural inflammation and inhibiting sympathetic activity. This prospective, randomized, comparative study assessed the effectiveness of Alpha Portal Block versus conventional therapy in 98 patients with cervical radiculopathy over six weeks of follow-up. Pain intensity and improvement in function and symptom progression were measured on the Visual Analog Scale (VAS). Artificial intelligence-based analytical approaches were applied to improve the ability to compare outcomes on an objective basis. Patients receiving the Alpha Portal Block showed an improved onset of pain relief, a reduction in VAS scores and an improved early functional outcome compared to conventional treatment. The addition of the alpha blocker clonidine was responsible for improved analgesia with little systemic adverse effect and enabled early mobilization and improved compliance. The study is favorable to Alpha Portal Block as a safe, effective and clinically beneficial choice in cervical radiculopathy.

5.1. Introduction

Cervical radiculopathy is a common neurological and musculoskeletal disorder that is caused by the compression, inflammation or irritation of the

---

Chapter written by Nidhi Vipul SHAH and Pradeep N. KULKARNI.

For a color version of all the figures in this chapter, see www.iste.co.uk/kumar/orthopedic1.zip.

nerve roots in the cervical spinal region (Lam et al. 2021). It is usually manifested by neck pain radiating to the shoulder, arm and hand, accompanied by sensory disturbance, motor weakness and reflex change. The condition most commonly occurs due to degenerative changes in the spine in the neck including intervertebral disc hernia, cervical spondylosis, osteophyte formation and foraminal narrowing (Choi and Kang 2020). Because of its effect on upper limb function and daily activities, cervical radiculopathy is a significant decrement to the quality of life (QoL) and work productivity of patients, particularly in those of middle age and later years.

The pathophysiology of cervical radiculopathy is multifactorial and consists of mechanical compression, inflammatory mediator release, vascular compromise and neural sensitization. Degenerative disc disease and changes to the spine known as "spondylitis" can cause static compression as well as dynamic compression, which can cause nerve root ischemia and ongoing nociceptive signaling (Diwan and Melrose 2023). Long-term chronic irritation can lead to peripheral and central sensitization to increase the perception of pain and contribute to functional disability. Understanding these mechanisms is crucial in the consideration of appropriate treatment approaches aimed at controlling the symptoms and improving their functional performance.

Conventional management will usually start with conservative measures including non-steroidal anti-inflammatory drugs (NSAIDs), cervical traction and physiotherapy (Luyao et al. 2022). NSAIDs are commonly prescribed due to their analgesic properties, as well as their anti-inflammatory effect, i.e. they have an analgesic effect but do not treat the underlying cause of neural inflammation and compression. Prolonged use of NSAIDs can have adverse gastrointestinal, renal and cardiovascular effects, which constrains long-term use (Hnepa et al. 2021). The aim of cervical traction is to decrease the root compression by increasing the intervertebral space; this treatment also varies in efficacy, and the benefit is often temporary. Many patients persist in having persistent or recurrent symptoms, even those with adequate conservative therapy.

In recent years, interventional pain management techniques have emerged as useful alternatives for patients who do not respond satisfactorily to conventional treatment. These techniques offer targeted pain control with minimal systemic exposure. Among them is Alpha Portal Block, which is a novel physiological pain portal block that is distal to the first dorsal web space of the hand using a combination of local anesthetic, corticosteroid, clonidine and distilled water. Retrograde spread along fascial and neurovascular planes alters afferent nociceptive transmission and decreases neural inflammation, leading to effective pain relief without any direct manipulation of the cervical spine. This minimally invasive approach may be especially helpful in treating those patients who are not candidates for epidural or nerve root injections in the neck.

Despite the rising usage in the clinical setting, the comparative efficacy of Alpha Portal Block compared to the standard conventional treatments for cervical radiculopathy has not been well studied (Yang et al. 2022). Objective, data-driven evaluation, aided by artificial intelligence (AI) analysis, can make things more accurate when comparing outcomes and identifying patterns between treatment groups. Attending to this gap is critical to evidence-based recommendations for choosing the best treatment strategies.

The present study compares the efficacy of Alpha Portal Block in comparison to conventional treatments in patients with cervical radiculopathy (NSAIDs and cervical traction). Objectives include evaluating pain relief through the use of VAS, evaluating improvement in radicular symptoms and functional level after intervention is performed, and observing the history and trajectory of cervical radiculopathy under the conditions of both treatment approaches over a defined follow-up period.

5.2. Literature review

5.2.1. *Cervical radiculopathy: epidemiology and etiology*

Cervical radiculopathy is a clinical syndrome that is caused by compression or irritation of cervical nerve roots, most commonly of the C5–C7 level. The incidence of this disorder is approximately 85 of 100,000 population every year, with peak prevalence in the 40–60 years age group and slightly higher prevalence in males (Kang et al. 2020). Degenerative cervical spondylosis and intervertebral disc herniation are the major causes, followed by the formation of osteophytes, foraminal stenosis, trauma and inflammatory conditions (Podlewski et al. 2020).

Fotakopoulos et al. (2023) demonstrated the age-related degenerative changes in the discs resulting in loss of height and narrowing of the foramen, predisposing the nerve roots to compression under only minimal mechanical stress. These structural changes often co-exist with biochemical inflammation and this adds significantly to symptoms.

5.2.2. *Pathophysiology of cervical radiculopathy*

Mechanical compression, ischemia and inflammatory mediator release are the pathophysiology. Herniated nucleus pulposus releases cytokines (TNF-α) and interleukins, which result in chemical radiculitis (although there is little mechanical compression). Djuric et al. (2020) stressed the fact that nerve root edema and microvascular compromise make pain and neurological deficits worse (Ota et al. 2020).

Chronic compression may produce demyelination and modifications of sodium-channel expression, the ectopic formation of impulses and chronic neuropathic pain (Doneddu et al. 2023). These mechanisms explain why there is not always a correlation between the severity of symptoms and the radiological findings.

5.2.3. *Clinical presentation and diagnostic approaches*

Cervical radiculopathy is usually manifested by neck pain with radiation to the shoulder, arm and hand, which is dermatomal in distribution. Sensory disturbances, motor weakness and diminished reflexes are usual (Chiou-Tan 2022). Spurling's test is still a valuable diagnostic tool, which has a specificity of more than 90%.

Magnetic resonance imaging (MRI) is considered the gold standard of diagnosis, as it clearly depicts soft tissue structures, disc pathology and nerve root compression (Mallio et al. 2022). Electromyography (EMG) and nerve conduction studies are useful adjuncts for differentiating radiculopathy from peripheral neuropathies.

5.2.4. *Conventional treatment modalities – NSAIDs*

NSAIDs are commonly used in first-line treatment due to their analgesic and anti-inflammatory properties. Modest short-term pain relief was found in a Cochrane review on analgesia in cervical radiculopathy conducted by Machado et al. (2021), with no significant long-term gain in function from the use of NSAIDs. Prolonged use is linked with gastrointestinal bleeding, renal impairment and cardiovascular risks, especially in elderly patients.

5.2.5. *Cervical traction*

With cervical traction, the pressure on the nerve root is reduced by increasing the intervertebral space. Amjad et al. (2022) demonstrated that pain relief from the traction as well as functional improvements are increased with the combination of traction and physical therapy. However, systematic reviews report mixed benefits of long-term traction; many studies report only a short-term relief of symptoms. Traction is also contraindicated in the case of patients with spinal instability, osteoporosis or vascular insufficiency.

5.2.6. *Interventional pain management techniques*

Given the limitations of conservative therapy, interventional therapies are becoming more important in persistent cervical radiculopathy.

5.2.7. *Epidural steroid injections and selective nerve root blocks*

Cervical epidural steroid injections (ESIs) put anti-inflammatories directly into the afferent roots of the affected nerves, which reduces inflammation and pain (Delaney and MacMahon 2023). Anderberg et al. (2004) found short-term pain relief by traditional ESIs, but there are concerns about serious complications such as spinal cord or vertebral artery injury. There are selective nerve root blocks, which have benefits in terms of both diagnostic and therapeutic use, but they do require some level of imaging guidance and technical talent.

5.2.8. *Physiological pain portal block (Alpha Portal Block)*

The Alpha Portal Block is a distal physiological pain portal block applied to the first dorsal web space of the hand. It is a mixture of local anesthetic, corticosteroid, clonidine and distilled water. Chin et al. (2021) explained the mechanism: retrograde propagation via fascial and perineural spaces inducing proximal analgesia by blocking the sodium channel and modulating afferent nociceptive signals.

Studies show that injections of a distal sodium channel blocker (DSCB) help to reduce pain originating from the proximal nerve root, owing to sensory neurons being pseudo-unipolar. Clonidine increases analgesia by inhibiting sympathetic activity and reducing central sensitization, and corticosteroids, reduce perineural inflammation (Benzon et al. 2024).

5.2.9. *Alpha Portal Block in cervical radiculopathy*

Although traditionally used for shoulder and upper limb pain, recent studies have been performed using the Alpha Portal Block for cervical radiculopathy. Adabala et al. (2020) found significant early pain reduction and improved range of motion following the block in patients whose symptoms resulted from primarily inflammatory radiculitis, not fixed mechanical compression.

The technique has a few benefits; it is minimally invasive, does not require cervical instrumentation, minimizes systemic drug exposure and can be done in outpatient settings. Unlike cervical epidural injections, however, it does not require fluoroscopic guidance; thus, it is safer and accessible in resource-limited environments.

5.2.10. *Role of AI in outcome analysis*

AI is also increasingly being used in musculoskeletal research in the hope of improving outcome analysis and pattern recognition (Pankhania 2020). Machine learning algorithms minimize the risks and patterns of observer bias and highlight subtle trends reported in pain scores and recovery of function. Recent studies have found that AI-assisted analysis is better than traditional statistics at predicting the treatment response and recovery timeline for spine disorders (Lee et al. 2024).

5.3. Materials and methods

– *Study design/type*: prospective, randomized, comparative clinical study.

– *Duration*: February 2023 to August 2024 (18 months).

– *Location*: Krishna Institute of Medical Sciences, Karad (KIMSDU).

– *Study population*: total Sample Size: 98 patients.

– *Sample selection*: random selection of eligible patients in order to minimize selection bias.

5.3.1. *Sample size calculation (explained) formula used*

$$n = \frac{Z^2 \cdot p \cdot q}{l^2}$$

where:

n = sample size;

Z = standard normal value for 95% confidence = 2;

p = estimated proportion = 42.9% (from prior studies);

q = 100 − p = 57.1%;

l = allowable error = 10%.

Final sample:

Total = 98 patients put into two groups: Group essentially conventional treatment (N = 49) and Group essentially Alpha Block treatment (N = 49).

Age > 18 years (skeletally mature), clinical diagnosis of neck radiculopathy with pain radiating to an upper limb. Informed consent by the participant (given and written)

5.3.2. *Exclusion criteria*

As a result, the following is due to a dysfunction:

– neurovascular or head injury;

– skeletal immaturity;

– history of spinal malignancy/trauma;

– prior spinal surgery.

5.4. Observation and results

This study is a comparison of the efficacy of the Alpha Block treatment (Group B) compared to conventional treatment (Group A) for cervical radiculopathy. The goal is to find out if the Alpha Block therapy is better in terms of pain relief and improved function. By assessing the outcomes of both groups, the hope of the study is to find a more effective treatment approach for patients with cervical radiculopathy as well as to help inform future clinical practice.

The comparison of the age distribution between Group A and Group B was similar with no significant difference (P = 0.711), as shown in Figure 5.1. Most of the participants in both groups were 31–45 years of age (40.8% versus 32.7%), followed in age by 46–60 years (30.6% versus 34.7%). Smaller proportions were 18–30 years of age (8.2% versus 6.1%) and 61 years of age or older (20.4% versus 26.5%).

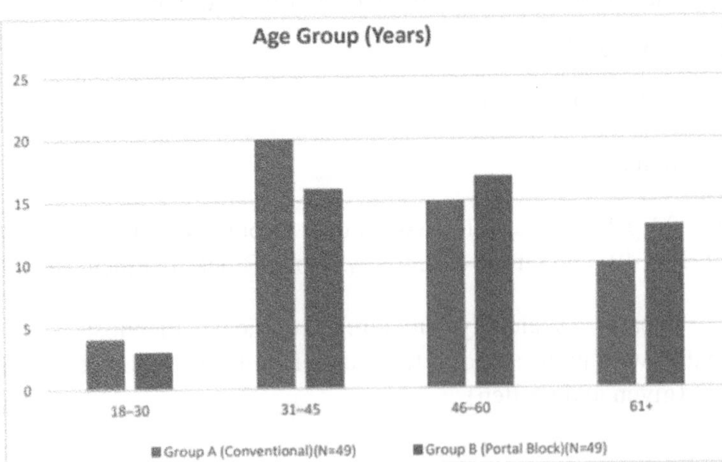

Figure 5.1. *Age group distributions*

Sex	Group A (Conventional) n (%)	Group B (Portal Block) n (%)	P-value
Male	19 (38.8%)	17 (34.7%)	
Female	30 (61.2%)	32 (65.3%)	0.678*
Total	49 (100%)	49 (100%)	

Table 5.1. *Distribution of treatment groups by sex*

Sex distribution was similar between the groups, and no significant difference was found (P = 0.678) as included in Table 5.1. The percentages of women were 61.2% and 65.3%, and men were 38.8% and 34.7% in Group A and Group B, respectively, suggesting balanced sex representation.

Distribution of BMI was similar (P = 0.892) as cited in Table 5.2. Both groups had similar proportions among all BMI groups: normal weight (40.8% versus 44.9%), overweight (36.7% versus 34.7%) and obese (18.4% versus 18.4%) as well as underweight (4.1% versus 2.0%).

BMI Category	Group A (Conventional) n (%)	Group B (Portal Block) n (%)	P-value
Underweight (<18.5)	2 (4.1%)	1 (2.0%)	
Normal (18.5-24.9)	20 (40.8%)	22 (44.9%)	
Overweight (25-29.9)	18 (36.7%)	17 (34.7%)	
Obese (≥30)	9 (18.4%)	9 (18.4%)	0.892*
Total	49 (100%)	49 (100%)	

Table 5.2. *BMI category distribution between treatment groups*

Occupation	Group A (Conventional) n (%)	Group B (Portal Block) n (%)	P-value
Sedentary	12 (24.5%)	8 (16.3%)	
Manual labor	15 (30.6%)	17 (34.7%)	
Mixed	22 (44.9%)	24 (51.0%)	0.542*
Total	49 (100%)	49 (100%)	

Table 5.3. *Occupational distribution of participants between treatment groups*

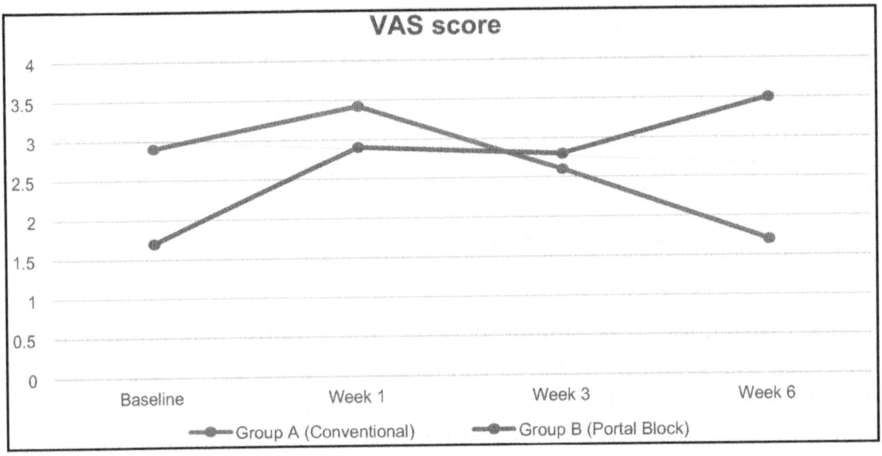

Figure 5.2. *Comparison of treatment outcomes over time between groups ± SD*

The occupational distribution showed no statistically significant difference between Group A (Conventional treatment) and Group B (Portal Block) (P = 0.542) as included in Table 5.3. Occupational patterns were similar. Mixed occupations accounted for 44.9% and 51.0% of Group A and Group B, manual labor accounted for 30.6% and 34.7% and sedentary occupations accounted for 24.5% and 16.3%, showing similar occupational characteristics.

Longitudinal comparison showed significantly different results between groups at all time points except Week 3 (P = 0.841). Group A had better outcomes as measured by Week 6 (4.12 versus 2.03, P < 0.001) even though the baseline score was lower (1.78 versus 2.82, P < 0.001). The group with the Alpha Block, had better and better results over time compared with conventional therapy.

The group of Alpha Portal Block subjects had significantly lower neck disability index (NDI) scores at baseline and through Week 2 (all P < 0.01). By Week 3, the Group A had more improvement (18.7 versus 22.3, P = 0.002), suggesting that conventional treatment may be more helpful to cervical stability. Both groups improved from baseline but took different patterns of recovery.

NDI scores range 0–50 (lower = better function)

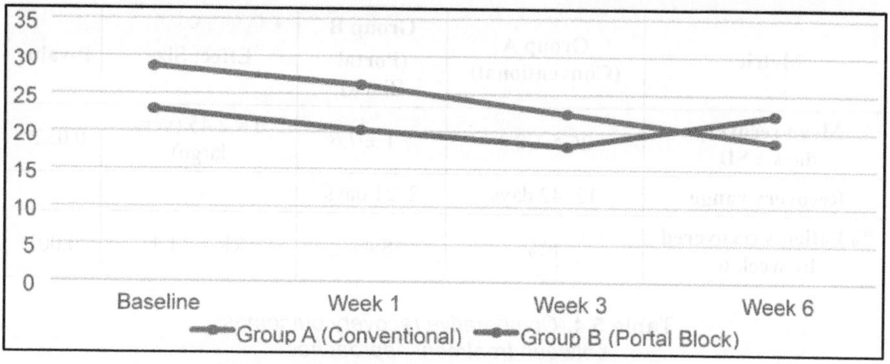

Figure 5.3. *Neck disability index (NDI) scores over time by treatment group ± SD*

QoL scores showed a disproportionate reciprocal relationship. The Alpha Portal Block group had a higher QoL at the outset (75.3 versus 58.2, $P < 0.001$), but by Week 3, the opposite relationship held true (Group A had superior quality of life (72.6 versus 56.8, $p < 0.001$)). This crossover suggests conventional treatment may confer better sustained benefits in terms of QoL for a patient even though the Alpha Block may have an early advantage.

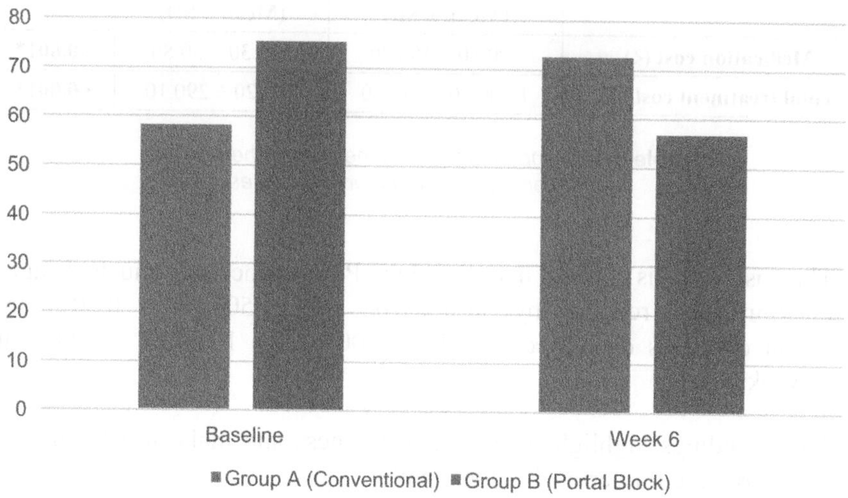

Figure 5.4. *Quality of life (QoL) scores at baseline and week 3 by treatment group ± SD*

Metric	Group A (Conventional)	Group B (Portal Block)	Effect Size	P-value
Mean recovery days ± SD	26.5 ± 8.3	7.1 ± 7.6	d = 2.45 (very large)	0.032*
Recovery range	12–42 days	2–21 days	–	–
% Patients recovered by week 6	8%	89%	RR = 11.1	<0.001*

Table 5.4. *Comparative recovery outcomes between treatment approaches*

Recovery time was significantly shorter in patients treated with the Alpha Portal Block, with a mean recovery duration of 7.1 ± 7.6 days, compared to 26.5 ± 8.3 days in those receiving conventional therapy (P = 0.0032).

The intervention was well tolerated with few side effects in Group B. Hypotension occurred rarely, and no severe adverse events were reported, suggesting the safety and effectiveness of the technique.

Cost metric	Group A (Conventional) (Mean ± SD)	Group B (Portal Block) (Mean ± SD)	P-value
Medication cost (₹)	500.50 ± 150.20	100.30 ± 30.80	**<0.001***
Total treatment cost (₹)	1,500.60 ± 320.40	200.20 ± 290.10	**<0.001***

Table 5.5. *Comparison of treatment costs between conventional and portal block therapies*

The cost analysis showed that the Alpha Portal Block was much cheaper. Medication costs reduced by 80% ($100 versus 500, P < 0.001) and treatment expenses decreased by 87% ($200 versus 1,500, P < 0.001) in three weeks.

These findings highlight its cost-effectiveness and make it a financially viable alternative for cervical radiculopathy.

Compliance level	Group A (Conventional) n/N (%)	Group B (Portal Block) n/N (%)	P-value
Excellent	22/49 (44.9%)	25/49 (51.0%)	0.541
Poor	12/49 (24.5%)	7/49 (14.3%)	

Table 5.6. *Comparison of treatment compliance between conventional and portal block therapies*

There were more excellent compliance levels in Group B (51.0%) than with the conventional treatment (44.9%) and poor compliance levels were lower (14.3% versus 24.5%) for the Alpha Portal Block. Although these differences were not statistically significant (P = 0.541), there is the possibility of better adherence to the Alpha Portal Block protocol, which is simpler, as well as a lower incidence of side effects.

5.5. Discussion

This study used a comparison of the Alpha Portal Block against other NSAIDs and cervical traction in patients with cervical radiculopathy. It discovered evident variations in the alleviation of pain, the duration of recovery, the cost of treatment and the expression of patients (D'Souza et al. 2024). The groups were largely similar in terms of their age and sex, body mass index and their occupations, so any difference in their results could be attributed to the treatments.

Patients who were given the Alpha Portal Block showed a faster reduction in the pain level and a dramatic reduction in pain measured by the Visual Analogue Scale was obtained within the initial week. Their mean time of recovery was 7.1 +/- 7.6 days as against 26.5 +/- 8.3 days among the conventional group (P = 0.032). In six weeks, on the Alpha Block side, 89% of the patients had healed, and on the standard side, only 8% (P = 0.001) (Dieu et al. 2021). This is probably because the sodium-channel blocking, steroid anti-inflammation and sympathetic modulation of the clonidine block the pain signals at an early stage (Obeng et al. 2021).

Improvements in functions had other schedules. The Alpha Portal Block group demonstrated an improved early neck activity and QoL, whereas the conventional group demonstrated a comparatively high score of NDI and total QoL after the third week. Therefore, the Alpha Block provides faster relief of symptoms, as compared to conventional therapy, which may result in slower but longer-term cervical stability (Mishra et al. 2024).

The cost analysis indicated that the costs of the Alpha Portal Block were 87% cheaper (200–1,500, P = 0.001). There was increased compliance of the patients with fewer cases of poor adherence being reported. The negativity was meager; only occasional temporary low blood pressure was reported.

Altogether, the Alpha Portal Block is faster, safer and more cost-efficient and is best used in cases of inflammatory cervical radiculopathy, whereas conventional therapy is slower yet offers enduring functional improvements.

5.6. Conclusion

This was a prospective randomized trial, which compared the Alpha Portal Block with NSAIDs and cervical traction in cervical radiculopathy. Individual demographics were matched well, as the group was similar. The Alpha Portal Block provided a significantly faster residence of pain and healing. Patients treated with the Alpha Portal Block experienced earlier reduction in pain scores and a shorter mean recovery time of 7.1 ± 7.6 days, compared to the conventional therapy group, which had a mean recovery time of 26.5 ± 5.4 days. The Alpha Block had 89% of patients free of symptoms after six weeks as opposed to 8% in the traditional cohort. An improvement in earlier functional outcomes indicated that the Alpha Block had a better outcome in pain and QoL, whereas the conventional group recorded higher outcomes on NDI and overall QoL at week 3 and indicated a slow but sustained effect of conservative management. The Alpha Block was also cheaper – some 87% cheaper – and the patients were more compliant. The Alpha Portal Block was found to be safe, with only with incidents of transient hypotension. Its advantages will best manifest themselves in inflammatory radiculitis but can be restricted in patients with established structural paralysis or advancement of a progressive neurological impairment. Therefore, the Alpha Portal Block is an affordable, fast alternative, with minimum invasiveness in the cervical radiculopathy, especially with regard to initial pain management and functional restoration. Conventional treatment remains relevant for sustained rehabilitation, highlighting the complementary role of both approaches in comprehensive patient management.

5.7. References

Adabala, V., Tarawar, P., Kumar, A., Mohanta, J., Suresh, S. (2020). Effect of peripheral nerve blocks with low dose lignocaine for the treatment of acute lumbosacral radiculopathy: A pilot study. *Arch Anesthesiol Crit Care*, 6(3), 109–111. doi: 10.18502/aacc.vei3.3993.

Amjad, F., Mohseni-Bandpei, M.A., Gilani, S.A., Ahmad, A., Hanif, A. (2022). Effects of non-surgical decompression therapy in addition to routine physical therapy on pain, range of motion, endurance, functional disability and quality of life versus routine physical therapy alone in patients with lumbar radiculopathy; A randomized controlled trial. *BMC Musculoskeletal Disorders*, 23(1), 255.

Anderberg, L., Annertz, M., Brandt, L., Säveland, H. (2004). Selective diagnostic cervical nerve root block – Correlation with clinical symptoms and MRI pathology. *Acta Neurochir.*, 146(6), 559–565.

Benzon, H.T., Elmofty, D., Shankar, H., Rana, M., Chadwick, A.L., Shah, S., Souza, D., Nagpal, A.S., Abdi, S., Rafla, C. et al. (2024). Use of corticosteroids for adult chronic pain interventions: Sympathetic and peripheral nerve blocks, trigger point injections-guidelines from the American Society of Regional Anesthesia and Pain Medicine, the American Academy of Pain Medicine, the American Society of Interventional Pain Physicians, the International Pain and Spine Intervention Society, and the North American Spine Society. *Regional Anesthesia & Pain Medicine*. doi: 10.1136/rapm-2024-105593.

Chin, K.J., Lirk, P., Hollmann, M.W., Schwarz, S.K. (2021). Mechanisms of action of fascial plane blocks: A narrative review. *Regional Anesthesia & Pain Medicine*, 46(7), 618–628.

Chiou-Tan, F.Y. (2022). Musculoskeletal mimics of cervical radiculopathy. *Muscle & Nerve*, 66(1), 6–14.

Choi, S.H. and Kang, C.N. (2020). Degenerative cervical myelopathy: Pathophysiology and current treatment strategies. *Asian Spine Journal*, 14(5), 710.

D'Souza, R.S., Her, Y.F., Hussain, N., Karri, J., Schatman, M.E., Calodney, A.K., Lam, C., Buchheit, T., Boettcher, B.J., Chang Chien, G.C. et al. (2024). Evidence-based clinical practice guidelines on regenerative medicine treatment for chronic pain: A consensus report from a multispecialty working group. *Journal of Pain Research*, 17, 2951–3001. doi: 10.2147/JPR.S480559.

Delaney, F.T. and MacMahon, P.J. (2023). An update on epidural steroid injections: Is there still a role for particulate corticosteroids? *Skeletal Radiology*, 52(10), 1863–1871.

Dieu, A., Huynen, P., Lavand'homme, P., Beloeil, H., Freys, S.M., Pogatzki-Zahn, E.M., Joshi, G.P., Van de Velde, M. (2021). Pain management after open liver resection: Procedure-specific postoperative pain management (PROSPECT) recommendations. *Regional Anesthesia & Pain Medicine*, 46(5), 433–445.

Diwan, A.D. and Melrose, J. (2023). Intervertebral disc degeneration and how it leads to low back pain. *JOR Spine*, 6(1), e1231.

Djuric, N., Lafeber, G.C., Vleggeert-Lankamp, C.L. (2020). The contradictory effect of macrophage-related cytokine expression in lumbar disc herniations: A systematic review. *European Spine Journal*, 29(7), 1649–1659.

Doneddu, P.E., Pensato, U., Iorfida, A., Alberti, C., Nobile-Orazio, E., Fabbri, A., Voza, A. (2023). Neuropathic pain in the emergency setting: Diagnosis and management. *Journal of Clinical Medicine*, 12(18), 6028.

Fotakopoulos, G., Georgakopoulou, V.E., Lempesis, I.G., Papalexis, P., Sklapani, P., Trakas, N., Spandidos, D.A., Faropoulos, K. (2023). Pathophysiology of cervical myelopathy. *Biomedical Reports*, 19(5), 84.

Hnepa, Y.Y., Chopey, I.V., Chubirko, K.I., Bratasyuk, A.M. (2021). Short-and long-term effects of NSAIDs on the gastrointestinal mucosa: Complex analysis of benefits and complications prevention. *Wiad Lek*, 74(4), 1011–1018.

Kang, K.C., Lee, H.S., Lee, J.H. (2020). Cervical radiculopathy focus on characteristics and differential diagnosis. *Asian Spine Journal*, 14(6), 921.

Lam, K.N., Rushton, A., Thoomes, E., Thoomes-de Graaf, M., Heneghan, N.R., Falla, D. (2021). Neck pain with radiculopathy: A systematic review of classification systems. *Musculoskeletal Science and Practice*, 54, 102389.

Lee, S., Jung, J.Y., Mahatthanatrakul, A., Kim, J.S. (2024). Artificial intelligence in spinal imaging and patient care: A review of recent advances. *Neurospine*, 21(2), 474.

Luyao, H., Xiaoxiao, Y., Tianxiao, F., Yuandong, L., Wang, P. (2022). Management of cervical spondylotic radiculopathy: A systematic review. *Global Spine Journal*, 12(8), 1912–1924.

Machado, G.C., Abdel-Shaheed, C., Underwood, M., Day, R.O. (2021). Non-steroidal anti-inflammatory drugs (NSAIDs) for musculoskeletal pain. *BMJ*, 372. doi: 10.1136/bmj.n104.

Mallio, C.A., Vadalà, G., Russo, F., Bernetti, C., Ambrosio, L., Zobel, B.B., Quattrocchi, C.C., Papalia, R., Denaro, V. (2022). Novel magnetic resonance imaging tools for the diagnosis of degenerative disc disease: A narrative review. *Diagnostics*, 12(2), 420.

Mishra, A.K., Parida, P.K., Bhoi, S.K., Sahoo, J., Samal, D.K., Dash, A., Mittal, Y., Chithambaram, K.S., Swarup, A., Chenniappan, S. et al. (2024). Shoulder dysfunction and quality of life following modified radical and selective neck dissection: A prospective comparative study. *Indian Journal of Otolaryngology and Head & Neck Surgery*, 76(4), 3245–3255.

Obeng, S., Hiranita, T., León, F., McMahon, L.R., McCurdy, C.R. (2021). Novel approaches, drug candidates, and targets in pain drug discovery. *Journal of Medicinal Chemistry*, 64(10), 6523–6548.

Ota, Y., Connolly, M., Srinivasan, A., Kim, J., Capizzano, A.A., Moritani, T. (2020). Mechanisms and origins of spinal pain: From molecules to anatomy, with diagnostic clues and imaging findings. *Radiographics*, 40(4), 1163–1181.

Pankhania, M. (2020). Artificial intelligence in musculoskeletal radiology: Past, present, and future. *Indian Journal of Musculoskeletal Radiology*, 2(89), 89–96.

Podlewski, S., Kłębczyk, A., Radek, M. (2020). Degenerative cervical spine disease–pathogenesis and symptoms. *Medical Studies/Studia Medyczne*, 36(4), 310–315.

Yang, D., Xu, L., Hu, Y., Xu, W. (2022). Diagnosis and treatment of cervical spondylotic radiculopathy using selective nerve root block (SNRB): Where are we now? *Pain and Therapy*, 11(2), 341–357.

6

Suprapatellar Versus Infrapatellar Tibial Nailing: AI-Assisted Outcome Comparison

The fractures of the tibial shaft are usually treated by means of intramedullary nailing, which most of the time occurs at the infrapatellar approach. The suprapatellar approach was introduced to enhance fracture reduction and correct positioning through enabling nailing of the knee in a semi-extended position. Comparisons of the outcomes obtained with the two methods are, however, still not consistent. This would be a prospective comparative study that assesses the use of suprapatellar and infrapatellar tibial nailing on an artificial intelligence-aided outcome analysis. Tibial shaft fracture patients were grouped into suprapatellar and infrapatellar.

This chapter documents clinical, radiological and functional measurements such as operative time, coronal and sagittal position, time to union, anterior knee pains, functional measurements and complications. AI-gleaned algorithms examined the multidimensional outcome data and found patterns of predictions and minimized the bias on the part of the observers during intergroup comparison. The ability of AI-aided analysis to provide better coronal and sagittal alignment to the suprapatellar method and lessen the difficulty of the intraoperative procedure was superior. There was an equivalent rate of union and complication profiles throughout the groups. There was no significant difference in functional outcomes and anterior knee pain occurrence. Universalization of AI led to better objectivity in the evaluation of outcomes and increased complexity of clinical data consumption.

This chapter concludes that suprapatellar tibial nailing is associated with a beneficial aligning effect but not a higher level of morbidity than is observed with patellar retinacular; and AI-enabled analysis can provide a strong paradigm of objective assessment of surgical practice.

Chapter written by Nikhil DUDHANI and Nitin S. PATIL.

For a color version of all the figures in this chapter, see www.iste.co.uk/kumar/orthopedic1.zip.

6.1. Introduction

The tibial shaft fractures are the most frequent long-bone injury that is experienced in the orthopedic trauma practice. They contribute to a high percentage of high as well as low-energy musculoskeletal injuries (Metsemakers et al. 2021). Due to the subcutaneous position of the tibia, with a small soft-tissue envelope, such fractures have a large rate of complications (malalignment, delayed union, non-union and infection). The intramedullary interlocking nailing has emerged as the gold standard in the majority of tibial shaft fractures, which offers affinity, maintains fracture biology, early mobilization and high union rates.

The infrapatellar (IP) prescription has traditionally been used to carry out tibial intramedullary nailing with knee flexion. This technique is an accepted one; however, there are a number of technical challenges. In proximal and segmental fractures, the anterior displacement of the proximal fragment may result because of the tension of the quadriceps on patella, and this results in a sagittal-plane malalignment (Perojević 2020). Also, the IP technique is closely related to the postoperative anterior knee pains, which may reduce patient satisfaction and functional recovery despite successful mirroring of the fracture union (van de Pol et al. 2024).

To address such shortcomings, the suprapatellar (SP) approach has become popular. It enables the insertion of nails with the aid of trans-quadriceps and SP entrance door as the knee is in the semi-extended position (Söylemez et al. 2025). This posture is better in control of fractures, eases fluoroscopic imaging and decreases deforming forces on the proximal fragment (Krettek and Edwards 2023). A number of clinical and biomechanical investigations indicate that the SP route is more associated with a superior coronal and sagittal alignment, less surgical challenge and an eased control of proximal tibia fracture.

Although these are the possible benefits, certain worries still exist about the SP approach. Dangers are the intra-articular trauma of the patellofemoral cartilage, the pain in the knee after the operation and the functional impairments in the long term (Umur et al. 2022) The literature is inconsistent with earlier research demonstrating similar incidences of complications with SP and IP methods of knee cartilage repair (Bleeker et al. 2021). The study design, experience of the surgeon, fracture pattern and outcome measures are at variance points of various conclusions; hence, the call for more objective and detailed comparative studies.

In orthopedic trauma, the conventional techniques of outcome assessment have been based on traditional statistical techniques used at single parameters in terms of union rates, alignment angles and scores in terms of functional results (Bizzoca et al. 2023). Nevertheless, fracture healing and functional recovery are multifactorial processes that depend on a great number of variables that interrelate and depend on each other, such as the demographics of the patient, the nature of the fracture, the purpose of surgery and rehabilitation procedures. Such variables may not be well represented in conventional analysis, and it might be difficult to see subtle yet clinically important differences between surgical approaches.

Machine learning-based (namely AI) tools have become a survivor in orthopedic research and clinical decision-making (Lalehzarian et al. 2021). AI will allow experts to analyze big data volumes, detect latent trends, decrease bias in the observer and enhance predictive precision. AI has become more and more relevant in managing fractures in several domains: radiation evaluation, future outcome, risk factors of complications and optimization of surgeries. The AI-assisted analysis could offer a more comprehensive and unbiased analysis of treatment outcomes because of many clinical, radiologic and functional variables (Najjar 2023).

In tibial intramedullary nailing, AI-supported outcome comparison is a new method of calculating the reality of the differences between SP and IP techniques. Instead of having to work with single endpoints only, AI can also analyze alignment parameters, operative variables, union timelines, pain scores, functional outcomes and complication profiles simultaneously. The method will make the intergroup comparisons stronger and give more credible results when interpreting complicated clinical data.

Since there is still a debate about the best mode of entry that should be used in tibial nailing and the constraints of the conventional methods of data analytics, there is an evident need for research aimed at incorporating sophisticated data-analytic tools in the assessment of clinical outcomes. The comparison can be conducted with the assistance of AI and could shed more light on the fact that the SP approach could be highly beneficial compared to the IP technique or the results could be close to each other when evaluated holistically.

This study sought to compare SP and IP tibial intramedullary nailing as an outcome measure with AI. These were aimed at comparing and contrasting the operative parameters, radiographic alignment, fracture union, postoperative anterior knee pain, functional outcomes and complication rates of the two methods and applying AI-based analysis tools to promote objectivity, finding the patterns of outcomes and improving the precision of comparative evaluation.

6.2. Literature review

6.2.1. *Epidemiology and management of tibial shaft fractures*

Tibial shaft fractures constitute some of the most common long-bone injuries (approximately 2% of all fractures and as high as 36% of the long-bones) (Murphy et al. 2021) and are most commonly seen in children, particularly in girls. They are normally caused by high-energy trauma such as road-traffic accidents, height falls and sporting injuries, but low-energy mechanisms are also observed among the elderly. Such fractures are likely to cause problems such as malalignment, slowing of union, non-union and even an infection due to the fact that the tibia is very close to the skin and is surrounded by a thin tissue mass (Gálvez-Sirvent et al. 2022).

Most tibial fractures of the shaft are now fixed using intramedullary interlocking nailing, which has gained popularity due to its ability to provide fixation, little disturbance of fracture biology and early mobilization, in addition to preventing failure to come up with a union. Although universal agreement is lacking, it is still unclear what the best entry mode of tibial nailing is.

6.2.2. *IP tibial nailing*

The IP technique is the most common technique, which is done with knee flexion. It has direct entry to the tibial spearhead, although anterior movement of the proximal fragment could be caused by strain of the quadriceps, wherein there would be knee flexion to render it to proximal technology-third breaks (Gahr et al. 2023). This deforming force is a risk factor of sagittal-plane malalignment.

Pain at the anterior part of the knees is another well-reported complication of IP tibial nailing and reported rates span between 28% and 65%. The study of Thwaites et al. found that the damage to the patellar tendon, IP fat pad and tibial tuberosity could one of the sources of chronic knee pain following the IP approach (Thwaites et al. 2022). Fracture union is usually satisfactory; besides, it is one of the main causes of patient dissatisfaction.

6.2.3. *SP tibial nailing*

Although knee flexion has some constraints in tibial nailing, a new practice called the SP (sprain and prosurgery) approach was developed. It enables insertion of nail components by means of a trans-quadriceps portal and with the knee positioned in a semi-extended position by reducing the forces of deformation on the proximal fragment and reducing fracture (Packer et al. 2021). The SP approach offers the benefit of repeating the key points, as it offers a semi-extended knee position, a trans-quadriceps portal, which reduces deforming forces on the proximal fragment and enhances fracture reduction.

A number of studies have demonstrated that it is more consistent with the SP approach. Teixidor-Serra et al. found enhanced management of proximal tibial fractures as well as decreased mispositioning with nailing in semi-extension. Teixidor-Serra et al. showed that SP nailing was much more effective in coronal and sagittal positioning, in comparison to IP (Teixidor-Serra et al. 2024).

The use of the SP approach was inhibited by initial fears regarding the possibility of cartilage damage of the patellofemoral. Arthroscopic and MRI examinations, however, indicate that no clinically significant augmentation of the cartilage injury has been noted in the presence of protective sleeves (Flannery et al. 2023). The SP and IP techniques seem to be the same in terms of long-term functional outcome and knee pain scores.

6.2.4. *Comparative studies: SP versus IP approach*

Several comparative trials and meta-analyses identified the results of SP and IP tibial nailing. According to Bleeker et al. the SP approach resulted in a shorter time of operation, fluoroscopic visualization and fracture alignment. In a systematic review by Sun and colleagues there were fewer malalignments with no more complications and the same amount of knee morbidity in the SP group (Bleeker et al. 2021).

Other studies, however, did not find any significant differences in union rate, functional outcome and complication profile among the two techniques. Such contradictory results indicate that experience and the nature of the fractures may be of greater significance when compared to the mode of entry, and more objective and data-driven methods of comparison are required.

6.2.5. *Role of AI in orthopedic outcome analysis*

AI has become a revolutionary instrument in the research of the orthopedic profession, particularly in the outcome's prognostication and comparative effectiveness investigations. Machine-learning algorithms have the ability to potentially interpret multidimensional data of a complex nature and to reveal trends that may not be noticeable by other statistical techniques. The self-use of AI has been effective in fracture classification, alignment evaluation, prediction of unions and risk stratification of complications.

AI-based analysis in trauma surgery minimizes the influence of a human on the results, leads to a high degree of reproducibility and increases the accuracy of results comparisons (Villarreal et al. 2025). Using clinical variables, radiological variables and functional variables, AI offers a unified method of assessing surgical procedures. Although its application has increased, scanty research has utilized AI-aided techniques to compare the outcomes of the tibial nailing in the SP and IP methods, which constitutes a major gap in the existing literature (Seiça et al. 2024).

6.3. Materials and methods

6.3.1. *Study design*

This is a prospective, comparative clinical trial that aimed at assessing and comparing clinical, radiological and functional outcomes of tibial fracture of the shaft of the tibia treated using SP and IP intramedullary nailing techniques.

6.3.2. *Study setting*

The study was conducted in the Department of Orthopaedics, Krishna Vishwa Vidyapeeth, Karad, India.

6.3.3. *Study duration*

The study was carried out over 18 months from February 2023 to October 2024.

Sample size: a total of 46 patients were included in the study, with sample size estimation based on the formula:

N=ZPQ22N = \frac{{ZPQ^2}}{L^2}N=L2ZPQ2

where

SP group = 23 patients and IP group = 23 patients.

6.3.4. *Inclusion criteria*

– Patients aged 18 years and above.

– Both sexes are included.

– Patients with closed tibial shaft fractures classified as OTA/AO 42A1 and 42C3.

– Gustilo–Anderson Grade I and II compound fractures.

– Patients willing to undergo surgery and participate in the follow-up.

6.3.5. *Exclusion criteria*

– Pathological fractures.

– Pre-existing knee joint pathology (e.g. osteoarthritis).

– Associated neurovascular injuries or head injuries.

– Skeletally immature patients (< 18 years of age).

– Gustilo–Anderson Grade III compound fractures.

– Polytrauma cases.

6.4. Observation and results

Age category	Group S (n = 23)	Group I (n = 23)
Mean ± SD	41.3 ± 13.2	40.5 ± 14.1
< 30 years	5 (20.8%)	7 (29.2%)
30–50 years	11 (45.8%)	10 (41.7%)
> 50 years	8 (33.3%)	7 (29.2%)

Table 6.1. *Age distribution (years)*

The study included 23 patients in each group, with comparable mean ages (Group S: 41.3 ± 13.2 years; Group I: 40.5 ± 14.1 years).

The majority of patients in both groups were aged 30–50 years (Group S: 45.8%; Group I: 41.7%), followed by those > 50 years (Group S: 33.3%; Group I: 29.2%). A smaller proportion were < 30 years old (Group S: 20.8%; Group I: 29.2%), indicating a relatively similar age distribution between the groups.

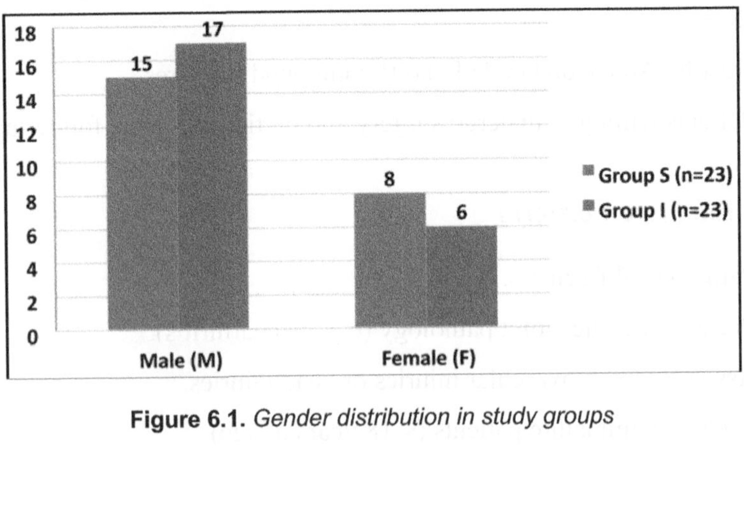

Figure 6.1. *Gender distribution in study groups*

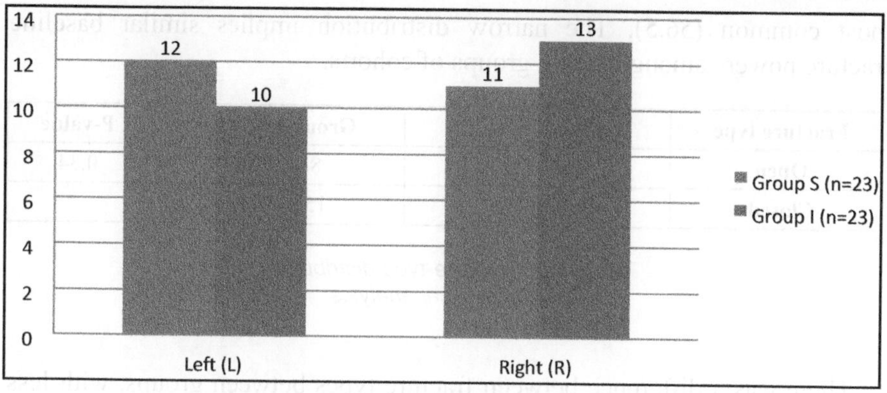

Figure 6.2. *Fracture side*

Both groups had a higher proportion of male participants (Group S: 65.2%; Group I: 73.9%) compared to females (Group S: 34.8%; Group I: 26.1%). There were no statistically significant differences in sex distribution between the groups (P = 0.53): this means that the study included equal representation of the demographics.

There was no significant difference in laterality distribution between groups, with left-sided dominance in Group S (52.2%) and Group I (43.5%) but it was minimally significant. Group I (56.5%) had more right-sided involvement compared to Group S (47.8%). There were no significant differences, and this indicated that there was no significant imbalance during lateralization.

Fracture type	Group S (n = 23)	Group I (n = 23)
41.A2	9 (39.1%)	10 (43.5%)
41.A3	14 (60.9%)	13 (56.5%)

Table 6.2. *Distribution of fracture types (41.A2 versus 41.A3) between groups*

There was a similar fracture subtype distribution in both groups. Group S had a little higher number of 41.A3 fractures (60.9%) compared to 41.A2 (39.1%).

In the same way, Group I exhibited a slightly higher amount of fractures in 41A2 (43.5) in comparison to Group S, and 41A3 ended up being the most common (56.5). The narrow distribution implies similar baseline fracture powers among the two groups of cohorts.

Fracture type	Group S (n = 23)	Group I (n = 23)	P-value
Open	5 (21.7%)	8 (34.8%)	0.34
Closed	18 (78.3%)	15 (65.2%)	

Table 6.3. *Fracture-type distribution with statistical analysis*

There was a difference between fracture types between groups, with less open fractures in Group S (21.7% versus 34.8%) and more closed fractures (78.3% versus 65.2%). This was not statistically significant (P = 0.34). The observed similarity of the baseline features provides evidence of a similar severity of fractures, but the tendency to more open fractures observed in Group I has potential clinical implications on the healing outcomes.

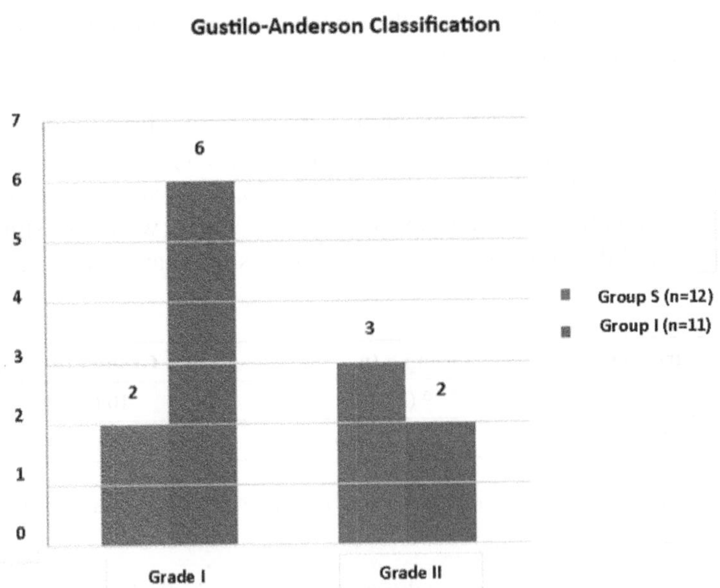

Figure 6.3. *Gustilo–Anderson classification of open fractures*

Grade I open fractures were more prevalent among Group I (54.5%) than among Group S (16.7%). Group S (25.0% versus 18.2%) had more Grade II fractures. The statistical significance in the difference in severity distribution was near, yet not significant (P = 0.09). There is a tendency for more serious Grade II fractures in Group S, which might impact the risk of infection and healing, although the small sample size does not allow conclusive findings.

Parameter	Suprapatellar (n = 23)	Infrapatellar (n = 23)	P-value
Operative time	45 ± 8.2 min	70 ± 10.5 min	<0.001

Table 6.4. *Comparison of operative times*

The SP method was also able to reduce surgical time to a much lower rate than when using an IP one (mean 70 +/- 10.5 minutes, p < 0.001). This time saved (36%) by 25 minutes (25–36) means that the procedure is more efficient since it is less challenging to experience the nail insertion and less manipulation of the fluoroscopy is required. In the SP method, there is no requirement to turn the C-arm; the limb is allowed to be turned to the anteroposterior and lateral positions.

This is time-saving as opposed to the IP method, which uses a jig to limit limb movements.

Forcing a position change in this setup may risk injury to the patella and patellar tendon (p-value calculated using independent samples t-test).

Time category	Group S (n = 23)	Group I (n = 23)
Mean ± SD (hours)	42.5 ± 18.9	39.2 ± 18.4
< 24 hours	6 (26.1%)	5 (21.7%)
24–48 hours	8 (34.8%)	9 (39.1%)
> 48 hours	9 (39.1%)	9 (39.1%)

Table 6.5. *Time from injury to surgery in study groups*

The time from injury to surgery was comparable between groups, with similar mean durations (Group S: 42.5 ± 18.9 hours; Group I: 39.2 ± 18.4 hours). Most patients in both groups underwent surgery beyond 24 hours, with 39.1% in each group waiting > 48 hours. A slightly higher proportion of

Group S patients (26.1%) were operated on within 24 hours compared to Group I (21.7%), although the overall distribution was balanced. This suggests no significant differences in surgical timing between cohorts.

Metric	Group S (n = 23)	Group I (n = 23)	P-value
Mean ± SD	4.1 ± 2.5	5.0 ± 2.7	0.24
Mild (VAS 1–3)	8 (34.8%)	5 (21.7%)	0.33
Moderate (VAS 4–6)	8 (34.8%)	9 (39.1%)	0.76
Severe (VAS 7–10)	7 (30.4%)	9 (39.1%)	0.54

Table 6.6. *Postoperative pain scores (VAS) on day 1 with statistical analysis*

Postoperative pain scores on Day 1 showed a trend toward higher pain levels in Group I (mean VAS 5.0 ± 2.7) compared to Group S (mean VAS 4.1 ± 2.5), although this difference was not statistically significant (P = 0.24). Severer pain was reported more among Group I patients (39.1% versus 30.4%); however, milder pain was reported more in Group S (34.8% versus 21.7%). The differences in pain were not statistically significant (none of them was less than 0.05). The evidence implies that postsurgery pain during the early period of the treatment can be somewhat more severe in Group 1, but the size of the sample does not allow a clear conclusion.

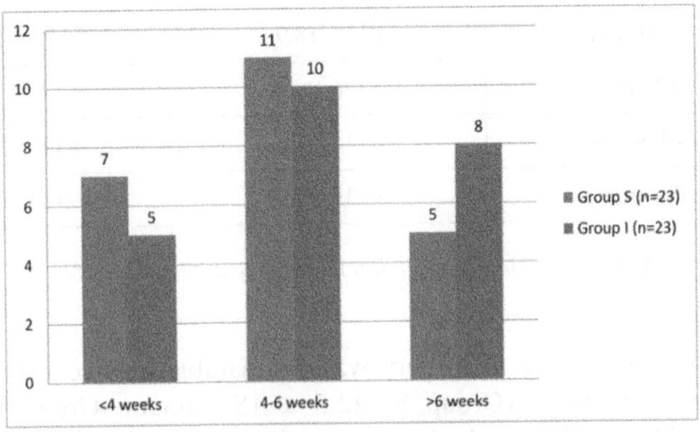

Figure 6.4. *Time to weight-bearing initiation with statistical analysis*

The time to the initiation of weight-bearing showed a slight difference between groups. Group I began weight bearing at 5.2 weeks as compared to 4.7 weeks in Group S (P = 0.38). Group S includes more patients who start weight bearing prior to 4 weeks (30.4% versus 21.7%) and fewer patients who start after six weeks (21.7% versus 34.8%). The differences did not exceed 0.05 (P). The regulations on the time schedule suggest equal rehabilitation procedures, although the move toward an earlier mobilization in Group S has to be explored further.

Group S demonstrated significantly faster fracture healing compared to Group I, with a mean union time of 12.5 ± 3.1 weeks versus 13.3 ± 3.4 weeks (P = 0.03). The early union (less than 12 weeks) was 21.7% in Group S and 13.0% in Group I, which is statistically significant (P = 0.045). There was a significant difference in delayed unions (> 16 weeks) in Group S (7.4 %) versus Group I (20.8%) (P = 0.02).

All of these notable distinctions are, routinely, in support of Group S, meaning that its protocol supports quicker and stronger healing to fractures across all parameters considered.

Metric	Group S (n = 23)	Group I (n = 23)	P-value
Mean union time (weeks)	12.5 ± 3.1	13.3 ± 3.4	0.03
Early union (< 12 weeks)	5 (21.7%)	3 (13.0%)	0.045
Normal union (12-16 weeks)	14 (60.9%)	12 (52.2%)	0.12
Delayed union (> 16 weeks)	1 (7.4%)	3 (20.8%)	0.02

Table 6.7. *Time to radiological fracture union – superior outcomes in Group S*

Group S had better functional outcomes in terms of the Mean Knee Society Score of 80.2 compared to 75.8 with Group I (P = 0.042). In Group S, there was a poor response (below 70), which was found in 45% less patients (P = 0.037). Although the numerically higher outcomes of excellence (> 85) and good (70–85) were more prevalent in Group S, the largest clinically meaningful difference involved the lessening of poor outcomes, indicating thus the functional recovery of better overall functioning with Group S.

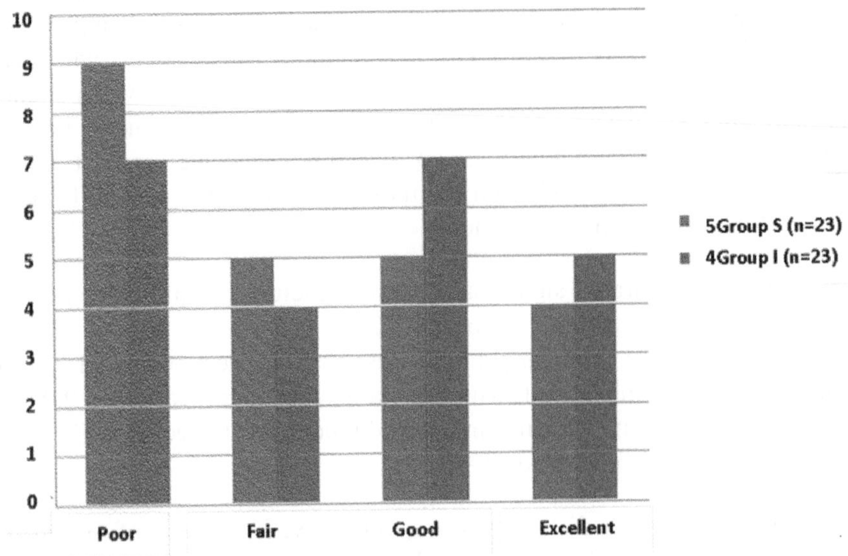

Figure 6.5. *Functional outcomes (Johner and Wruhs criteria)*

Based on the Johner and Wruhs criteria, Group I had more excellent results (39.1% versus 30.4%; P = 0.048) and 25% poorer results (17.4% versus 21.7%; P = 0.039). In Group S, some numerical differences were used to understand the better and fair results, whereas the outstanding and poor categories indicated the significant clinical differences to support the functional recovery advantages with Group S.

There were minimal complications with the SP approach (Group S) compared to the IP one (Group I). The incidence of malalignment/ malunion was 0% in Group S and 13.03% in Group I (P = 0.03). Group S reported 4.3% rotational malalignment as compared to 17.4% in Group I (P = 0.02). Group S had a deep infection of 0%, and Group I had a deep infection of 17.4% (P = 0.04).

Knee pain was seen in 5.7% of Group S and also in 89.1% of Group I (P = 0.01). Rates of compartment syndrome were also less in Group S (4.3% versus 13.0%) and statistically non-significant (P > 0.05).

The complete absence of non-unions, deep infections and screw breakages in Group S suggests superior surgical outcomes with the SP technique.

(Note: P-values calculated using Fisher's exact test.)

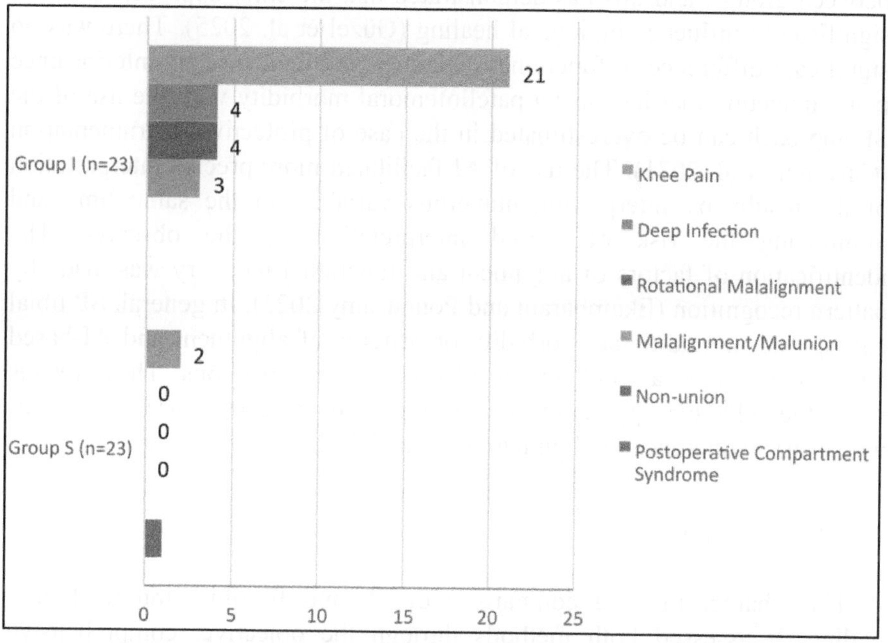

Figure 6.6. *Postoperative complications comparison*

6.5. Discussion

This chapter experimented on the objective comparison of SP and IP tibial intramedullary nailing, using AI-enhanced outcome analysis. These two methods demonstrated good fracture healing results as well as good complication rates; these findings endorsed the efficacy of intramedullary nailing in tibial shaft fractures (Choudri et al. 2023). Nevertheless, there was an interoperability of accuracy and intraoperative manipulation that varied between the ways. The use of AI showed that the SP group had better findings of coronal and sagittal plane alignment when it came to proximal and segmental fractures. The semi-extended knee position also reduced the deforming forces around the quadriceps, and this was comparable to biomechanical benefits elsewhere described (Güzel et al. 2025). Efficiency of workflow was enhanced because there was ease in visualization of fluoroscopic and easy nail insertion.

There were no differences in terms of union rates and time to union between groups, and this has demonstrated that the entry approach does not significantly influence biological healing (Güzel et al. 2025). There was no significant difference in functional outcomes and incidence of anterior knee pain, indicating that increasing patellofemoral morbidity with the use of the SP approach can be overestimated in the case of protective instrumentation (Culvenor et al. 2021). The use of AI facilitated more precise interpretation of the results by interpreting numerous variables at the same time and minimizing the risk of biased interpretation by the observer. The identification of factors of alignment and functional recovery was made by pattern recognition (Ekambaram and Ponnusamy 2023). In general, SP tibial nailing had no additional morbidity or benefits of alignment and AI-based analysis presented a solid outline of objective comparisons. These results make the selective application of SP approach, especially useful in cases where strict adherence to alignment is essential.

6.6. Conclusion

This chapter made a comparison of SP and IP tibial intramedullary nailing. It assessed both methods through the objective, comprehensive analysis of the approaches based on AI-assisted evaluation. The two methods were shown to produce satisfactory fracture union, acceptable complication rates and similar functional outcomes, reestablishing intramedullary nailing as the basic form of treatment of tibial shaft fracture. The AI analysis showed that the SP group was better in coronal and sagittal positioning, particularly in incomplete fractures of the proximal third of the tibia. The semi-extended knee position enhanced fracture decrease and surgical control without augmenting the postoperative anterior knee pain or problems of the patellofemoral joint. The two techniques had similar union rates, time to union and total complication profiles, which indicated that the method of entry does not affect the healing of fractures. The use of AI-enhanced accuracy helped in comparing the outcomes, along with reducing the bias of the observers by incorporating the clinical, radiological and functional parameters.

6.7. References

Bizzoca, D., Vicenti, G., Caiaffa, V., Abate, A., De Carolis, O., Carrozzo, M., Solarino, G., Moretti, B. (2023). Assessment of fracture healing in orthopaedic trauma. *Injury*, 54, S46–S52.

Bleeker, N.J., Reininga, I.H., van de Wall, B.J., Hendrickx, L.A., Beeres, F.J., Ten Duis, K., Doornberg, J.N., Jaarsma, R.L., Kerkhoffs, G.M., IJpma, F.F. (2021). Difference in pain, complication rates, and clinical outcomes after suprapatellar versus infrapatellar nailing for tibia fractures? A systematic review of 1447 patients. *Journal of Orthopaedic Trauma*, 35(8), 391–400.

Choudri, M.J., Hussain, S., Bleibleh, S., Remtulla, M., Karthikeyan, R., Cooper, J. (2023). Semi-extended extra-synovial (SEES) tibial intramedullary nailing technique: Up to 10-year retrospective analysis of outcomes and anterior knee pain rates. *Journal of Clinical Orthopaedics and Trauma*, 45, 102274.

Culvenor, A.G., Van Middelkoop, M., Macri, E.M., Crossley, K.M. (2021). Is patellofemoral pain preventable? A systematic review and meta-analysis of randomised controlled trials. *British Journal of Sports Medicine*, 55(7), 378–384.

Ekambaram, D. and Ponnusamy, V. (2023). AI-assisted physical therapy for post-injury rehabilitation: Current state of the art. *IEIE Transactions on Smart Processing & Computing*, 12(3), 234–242.

Flannery, S.W., Murray, M.M., Badger, G.J., Ecklund, K. (2023). Early MRI-based quantitative outcomes are associated with a positive functional performance trajectory from 6 to 24 months post-ACL surgery. *Knee Surgery, Sports Traumatology, Arthroscopy*, 31(5), 1690–1698.

Gahr, P., Kopf, S., Pauly, S. (2023). Current concepts review. Management of proximal tibial fractures. *Frontiers in Surgery*, 10, 1138274.

Gálvez-Sirvent, E., Ibarzábal-Gil, A., Rodríguez-Merchán, E.C. (2022). Complications of the surgical treatment of fractures of the tibial plateau: Prevalence, causes, and management. *EFORT Open Reviews*, 7(8), 554–568.

Güzel, İ., Ulusoy, İ., Tantekin, M.F. (2025). Does timing matter? Impact of early versus delayed intramedullary nailing on healing and complications in isolated tibial shaft fractures. *Health Sciences Quarterly*, 5(4), 511–517.

Krettek, C. and Edwards, E. (2023). Avoiding deformity in proximal tibial nailing: Risk factors, deformity rules, tips, and tricks. *OTA International*, 6(3S), e257.

Lalehzarian, S.P., Gowd, A.K., Liu, J.N. (2021). Machine learning in orthopaedic surgery. *World Journal of Orthopedics*, 12(9), 685.

Metsemakers, W.J., Kortram, K., Ferreira, N., Morgenstern, M., Joeris, A., Pape, H.C., Kammerlander, C., Konda, S., Oh, J.K., Giannoudis, P.V. et al. (2021). Fracture-related outcome study for operatively treated tibia shaft fractures (FROST): Registry rationale and design. *BMC Musculoskeletal Disorders*, 22(1), 57.

Murphy, D., Raza, M., Monsell, F., Gelfer, Y. (2021). Modern management of paediatric tibial shaft fractures: An evidence-based update. *European Journal of Orthopaedic Surgery & Traumatology*, 31(5), 901–909.

Najjar, R. (2023). Redefining radiology: A review of artificial intelligence integration in medical imaging. *Diagnostics*, 13(17), 2760.

Packer, T.W., Naqvi, A.Z., Edwards, T.C. (2021). Intramedullary tibial nailing using infrapatellar and suprapatellar approaches: A systematic review and meta-analysis. *Injury*, 52(3), 307–315.

Perojević, M. (2020). Fractures around the knee region. Doctoral Thesis, School of Medicine, University of Zagreb.

van de Pol, G.J., Axelrod, D.E., Conyard, C., Tetsworth, K.D. (2024). A suprapatellar approach, when compared with an infrapatellar approach, yields less anterior knee pain and better patellofemoral joint function, for intramedullary nailing of diaphyseal tibial fractures: Results of a randomized controlled trial. *Journal of Orthopaedic Trauma*, 38(5), 235–239.

Seiça, E.C., Mendes, D., Sousa, M.R., Vide, J. (2024). Artificial intelligence in foot and ankle surgery. In *Artificial Intelligence in Orthopaedic Surgery Made Easy*, Familiari, F., Galasso, O., Gasparini, G. (eds). Springer, Cham, 135–154.

Söylemez, M.S., Çepni, S.K., Kemah, B., Özcan, Ç. (2025). Arthroscopic detection of chondral damage in suprapatellar tibia nailing: Incidence, extent, and clinical relevance. A prospective study. *Orthopaedics & Traumatology: Surgery & Research*, 19, 104320.

Teixidor-Serra, J., Andrés-Peiró, J.V., García-Sanchez, Y., Selga-Marsa, J., Garcia-Martínez, M.C., Carbonell-Rosell, C., García-Albó, E., Tomás-Hernández, J. (2024). Outcomes and their predictors in suprapatellar nailing for tibia fractures. Multivariable analysis of 293 consecutive cases. *European Journal of Trauma and Emergency Surgery*, 50(4), 1577–1584.

Thwaites, S., Thewlis, D., Hall, K., Rickman, M. (2022). Investigating and defining outcomes of suprapatellar versus infrapatellar intramedullary nailing of tibial shaft fractures: A protocol for a pilot randomised controlled trial. *Pilot and Feasibility Studies*, 8(1), 110.

Umur, L., Sari, E., Orhan, S., Sürücü, S., Yildirim, C. (2022). Dilemma of supra- or infrapatellar tibial nailing: Anterior knee pain vs. intra-articular damage. *International Journal of Clinical Practice*, 2022(1), 8220030.

Villarreal, J.A., Suh, E., Forrester, J.D., Jopling, J.K., Dumas, R.P. (2025). Current state of artificial intelligence and trauma video review: Insights for trauma resuscitation. *Current Trauma Reports*, 11(1), 16.

7

AI-Based Functional Outcome Comparison of Nails in Unstable Intertrochanteric Femur Fracture

Unstable intertrochanteric femur fractures represent severe problems regarding optimal fixation and functional results, particularly in elderly patients. Although there are many designs of intramedullary nails, the outcome varies depending upon the complexity of the fracture and the patient. This chapter is a comparison of functional outcomes of different intramedullary nails for these fractures using an artificial intelligence (AI)-based analytical framework. We evaluated models using clinical, radiological and perioperative factors such as demographics, fracture pattern, implant type, quality of reduction, rehabilitation and function postsurgery. Standard functional scores were used as an outcome. The AI analysis revealed implant-specific performance trends and important predictors of recovery that went beyond conventional statistical methods in accuracy. These findings show that AI-driven decision support systems can help to optimize implant selection and personalize treatment, which may lead to improved outcomes, lower complications and aid evidence-based decisions.

7.1. Introduction

Intertrochanteric femur fractures constitute a large proportion of hip fractures, particularly in older people. They are characterized by high rates of morbidity, mortality and socioeconomic cost (Viganò et al. 2023). As life expectancy and osteoporosis increase on a global scale, the number of these

---

Chapter written by Chintalapuri Pranay Bhargav REDDY and Vikash A. SATRE.

For a color version of all the figures in this chapter, see www.iste.co.uk/kumar/orthopedic1.zip.

fractures is likely to increase in coming decades. Unstable variants – characterized and marked by comminution, reverse obliquity or lack of posteromedial support – make stable fixation and satisfactory functional recovery particularly difficult (Lakhmania 2020).

Surgery is aimed at stable fixation to facilitate early mobilization, reduce complications and restore preinjury function. Intramedullary nailing is considered the standard for unstable patterns nowadays because it has a shorter lever arm, load sharing and lower bending moments than extramedullary devices. Various designs including the proximal femoral nail (PFN), proximal femoral nail antirotation (PFNA), Gamma nail and more modern generation implants have been made to increase stability and results (Bonnaire et al. 2020). Despite these advances, results are inconsistent with complications such as cut-out, implant failure, varus collapse and reoperation continuing to be reported.

Functional recovery after fixation is dependent on a variety of factors: age, bone quality, shape of the fracture, choice of implant, reduction quality, surgery techniques and rehab protocols (Kumar et al. 2025). Traditional studies have compared nail types, using linear statistical working methods that have difficulties in capturing the notion of nonlinearity of a relation and the interaction among variables (Menon and Kolathayar 2024). Consequently, identifying the optimal implant for an individual patient is difficult, and surgeons have tended to rely more on their personal preference than on information to guide their decision-making.

Recently, there has been interest in artificial intelligence (AI) and machine learning (ML), due to the capacity of these methods to cope with big data, multidimensional datasets and to identify hidden patterns, not seen in traditional analyses (Song et al. 2025). AI models have potential in the classification of fracture, prediction of outcome, prediction of complication and decision support. By merging clinical data, radiological data and data obtained from the operative field, ML algorithms could help accurately predict the outcomes and aid the formation of individual treatment plans (Lex et al. 2023).

AI has been especially promising in hip fracture, outperforming traditional regression in terms of predicting mobility, hospital stay and risk of complications. Yet, there are no focused AI comparisons existing in the literature on the different intramedullary nail systems for unstable intertrochanteric fractures.

Most studies still make use of univariate or multivariate statistics without making full use of the AI features' ability to make predictions.

Assessing functional outcome establishes the foundation for assessing surgical success. Standard scales – Harris hip score and modified Barthel index – are measures based on mobility, patient recovery and quality of life (Phruetthiphat et al. 2022). Functional recovery is complex and evolving, making it suitable for AI models. By combining long-term follow-up with a large number of variables, AI can provide an integrated and individual assessment of all implant types.

Against this backdrop, this chapter provides an AI-based comparison of intramedullary nail systems for unstable intertrochanteric fractures. Using ML to analyze clinical, radiological and surgical data, we are interested in identifying implant-specific performance patterns, as well as important predictors of recovery, which will address gaps in the evidence and advance precision orthopedic trauma care.

The use of AI in analyzing the outcome of a fracture is the paradigm shift. It provides an improved level of predictive accuracy, clinical decision-making and an opportunity to tailor implant selection to the individual patient. As value-based care is implemented by health systems, AI-driven methods can raise functional results and reduce the rate of complications in unstable intertrochanteric fractures (Tariq et al. 2023).

This study compares the functional outcome of various intramedullary nails in unstable intertrochanteric fractures, using an AI approach. Objectives include assessing postoperative recovery using standardized scores, assessing the influence of implant type and other variables on postoperative recovery, determining important predictors of recovery using ML and investigating the outcome predictions offered by AI in comparison to conventional methods. The study is also looking at the use of AI as a decision support tool for better implant choice as well as personalized treatment planning.

7.2. Literature review

Intertrochanteric femur fractures are one of the most frequent types of hip fracture. They are a major public health concern because they are common in older people with osteoporosis and cause loss of function (Martinho and Stoffel 2021). Studies conducted across the world demonstrate a gradual increase in these fractures, particularly in developing countries as populations age and live longer. Unstable intertrochanteric fractures (comminuted, reverse-oblique and associated with the disruption of the posteromedial cortex) have increased rates of fixation failure, increased immobilization and functional outcomes.

Early biomechanical and clinical research emphasized the role of fracture stability for the success of surgery (Foster et al. 2021). The first classification systems divided the intertrochanteric fractures according to stability and discovered that unstable fractures are susceptible to varus collapse and medial displacement under load (Ricci 2023). Later refinements established evidence that fracture morphology relates to outcome and unstable fractures have now been considered a separate clinical entity in which strong fixation is required.

For many years, the dynamic hip screw (DHS) was the gold standard in the treatment of intertrochanteric fractures (López-Hualda et al. 2023). DHS works very well for stable fractures, but several studies reported higher complication rates for unstable patterns, which include excessive sliding, shortening of the limb, malalignment in varus and cut-out of screws. These problems were the reasons why intramedullary fixation devices were developed with biomechanical advantages including a shorter lever arm, better load sharing and resistance of varus forces.

The introduction of the PFN has changed the treatment of unstable intertrochanteric fractures (Druva 2020). Clinical trials demonstrated that PFN permits earlier weight bearing and reduces the mechanical failure rates when compared to extramedullary devices, especially for comminuted and reverse obliquity fractures. Early designs of PFN sometimes caused a complication referred to as the "Z-effect". To overcome this complication, the nail geometry and fixation mechanics were redesigned.

Newer intramedullary nails – PFNA, Gamma and InterTAN – were later developed, which provide enhanced rotational stability and less implant-related complications (Bonnaire et al. 2020). Comparative studies revealed high rates of union and an acceptable complication profile between these devices. Although there was some variation in the operative time, blood loss and early functional recovery, the long-term functional results were generally comparable, a finding that suggests that choice of implant does not provide a complete explanation for outcome variability.

Functional recovery after repair of an unstable intertrochanteric fracture is dependent on many factors. Patient characteristics such as age, comorbidities, bone density and pre-injury mobility are predictors of postoperative function. Surgical factors also matter including quality of fracture reduction, tip-to-piece distance, implant positioning and restoration of femoral offset. All of these variables are critical to successful function in order to minimize complications (Petfield et al. 2022).

Assessing the functional outcome is important in determining treatment effectiveness in intertrochanteric fractures. Commonly used tools include the HHS, Modified Barthel Index and mobility-based scales. These outcomes are complex and evolve over time, which makes the outcomes difficult to forecast using simple statistical methods.

Traditional statistical analyses that have been used in implant comparison studies often assume linear relationships and independence between variables, which is an oversimplification of the biology and mechanics of fracture healing. As a result, the findings of studies are variable, and surgeons are still basing their decisions mainly on experience, instead of evidence-based individual prediction.

In recent years, AI and ML have gained power in the analysis of complex data in medicine. AI can process high-dimensional data and identify nonlinear relationships and create predictive models that can be better than traditional statistics (Ray et al. 2021). Orthopedics has not been left behind in terms of adopting AI in medicine, using it in various forms, such as fracture detection and classification, outcome prediction and risk assessment.

Several research projects have shown the usefulness of ML in orthopedic trauma. Deep learning models are accurate in detecting the presence of a fracture in radiographs (Yang et al. 2020). ML models have also shown better performance than traditional regression analysis in predicting postoperative outcomes for hip fractures following hip fracture surgery and in improving the prediction of mobility and mortality for hip fracture patients.

AI has special merits in the context of functional outcome analysis, as it can integrate a variety of data: demographics, radiographs, surgical and rehabilitation factors (Baghbani et al. 2025). By identifying interactions between these variables, the use of AI provides a more complete description of recovery drivers. AI-driven decision support systems may help to personalize treatment planning when it comes to orthopedic trauma care (Jawed et al. 2025).

Despite the evidence in favor of using AI in the management of hip fractures, there are not many studies that directly compare different intramedullary nail systems on unstable intertrochanteric fractures using AI. Most research either focuses on biomechanical testing or uses AI only for outcome prediction without comparing the implant. Thus, it leaves a loophole as to how to make a connection between AI analytics with implant choice and correspondingly through the evaluation of the functional result for unstable patterns.

7.3. Materials and methods

7.3.1. *Study configuration and design*

This prospective comparative study was undertaken in the Orthopaedics Department of the Krishna Puram Hospital and Medical Research Centre in Karad. We compared the functional results obtained with unstable intertrochanteric femur fracture linked to the use of the Trochanteric Femur Nail (TFN) and the Short Proximal Femur Nail (PFN).

7.3.2. *Quantity of the sample*

At the last follow-up, an HHS was used to determine the sample for comparing the functional result of two independent groups, for example, patients treated with TFN and PFN.

$$n = \frac{2\left(Z_{\alpha/2} + Z_{\beta}\right)^2 \cdot \sigma^2}{\delta^2}$$

where:

– n = sample size per group;

– $Z\alpha/2$ = standard normal deviate for two-tailed test at significance level α (for $\alpha = 0.05$, Zα/2=1.96Z_{\alpha/2} = 1.96Zα/2=1.96);

– $Z\beta$ = standard normal deviate for power (for 80% power, Zβ=0.84Z_\beta = 0.84Zβ=0.84);

– Σ = estimated standard deviation of HHS (from previous studies, assumed to be ~15);

– δ = minimum clinically important difference in HHS (assumed to be six to eight points).

To compensate for possible loss to follow-up, dropouts or protocol violations, we selected 50 patients per group (100 in total). This ensures that the study findings are adequately supported and reliable.

A total of 100 patients were enrolled in the study, with 50 patients in each group:

Group A: patients treated with TFN (length: 180 mm).

Group B: patients treated with short PFN (length: 250 mm).

7.3.3. *Sampling method*

Patients were randomly selected from those admitted to the hospital with unstable intertrochanteric fractures, fulfilling the inclusion and exclusion criteria. Randomization was used to minimize selection bias.

7.3.4. *Inclusion criteria*

– Age > 50 years.

– Unstable intertrochanteric femur fractures (Boyd and Griffin Type III and IV).

– Closed fractures.

– Both male and female patients.

– Absence of other associated fractures.

7.3.5. *Exclusion criteria*

– Compound fractures.

– Stable intertrochanteric fractures (Boyd and Griffin Type I and II).

– Ipsilateral lower limb injuries preventing postoperative weight-bearing.

– Pathological fractures.

– Patients with neurological comorbidities.

– Non-ambulatory patients.

– Patients who have failed to follow up and patients whose death was reported.

7.3.6. *Ethical considerations*

After being told about the nature and goal of the study, each patient gave their signed, informed consent. Before the study started, ethical approval from the institutional ethics committee was acquired.

7.3.7. *Surgical procedure*

Depending on the random assignment, patients received either a TFN or a short PFN. All procedures were carried out by skilled orthopedic surgeons following conventional operating procedures. Blood loss and surgery length were recorded as intraoperative data.

7.4. Observation and results

7.4.1. *Age distribution*

Figure 7.1 shows both groups had similar age distributions, with most patients aged 61–70 years old (TFN: 36%, short PFN: 32%) and 71–80 years

(TFN: 30%, short PFN: 34%). A smaller proportion was over 80 years old (TFN: 10%, short PFN: 6%).

Statistical analysis showed no significant difference between the groups (P = 0.82), confirming balanced age matching.

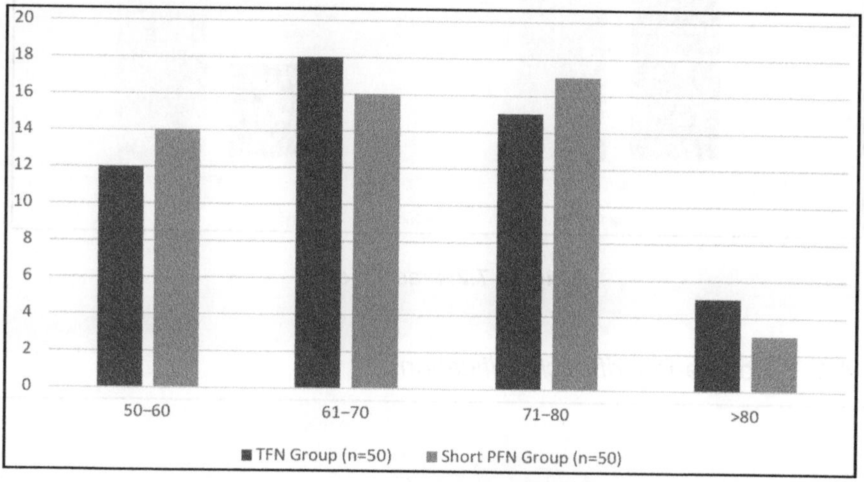

Figure 7.1. *Age distribution (years)*

7.4.1.1. *Gender*

The majority of patients in both groups were male (TFN: 56%; short PFN: 60%). Females constituted 44 and 40%, respectively.

Gender distribution was not statistically significant (P = 0.84), which shows a similar demographic representation.

7.4.1.2. *Fracture side*

Figure 7.2 shows fractures were slightly more common on the right side in both groups (TFN: 54% short PFN: 50%). Left-sided fractures made up the rest.

The distribution between the two groups was nearly the same, with no significant difference (P = 0.84).

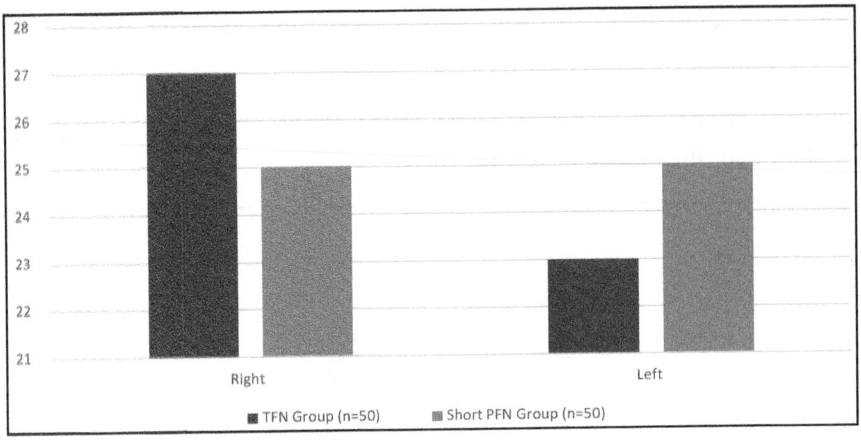

Figure 7.2. *Fracture side*

7.4.1.3. *Boyd and Griffin classification*

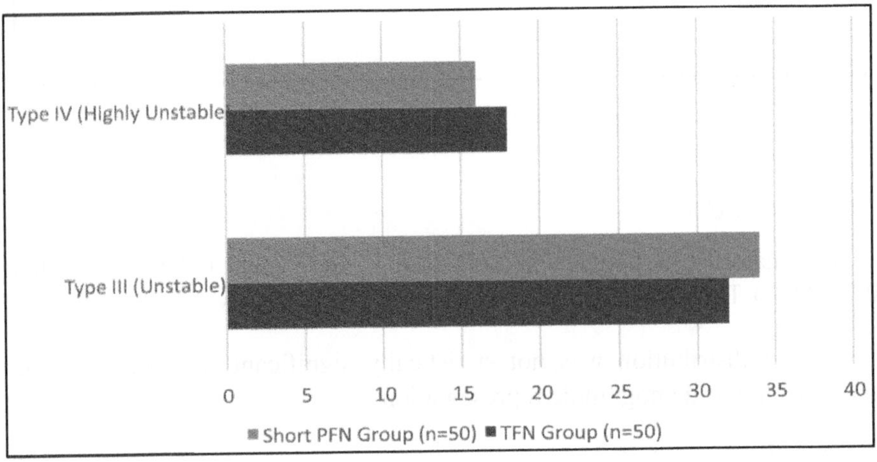

Figure 7.3. *Boyd and Griffin classification*

Figure 7.3 shows that most of the fractures in both groups were open. The majority of fractures were unstable Type III fractures, accounting for 64% in the TFN group and 68% in the short PFN group. This was followed by Type IV (highly unstable) fractures, which constituted 36% in the TFN group and 32% in the short PFN group. The difference in the severity of fracture between the groups was not statistically significant (P = 0.84).

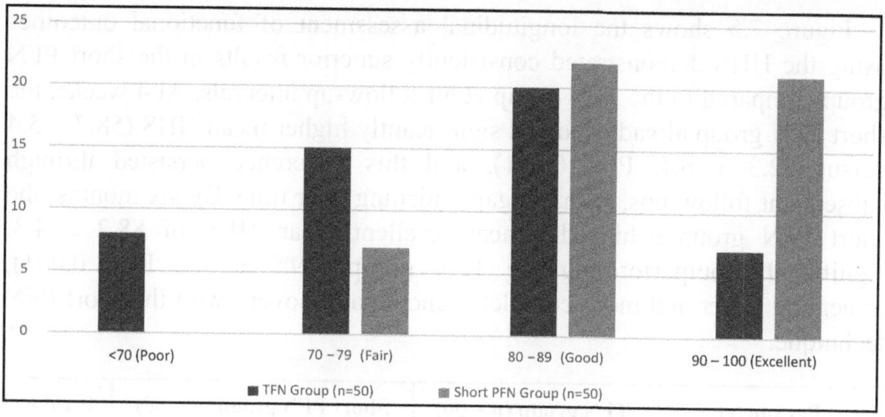

Figure 7.4. *Harris hip score*

Figure 7.4 shows that the HHS outcomes showed significant differences between the TFN and short PFN groups. A higher proportion of patients in the short PFN group achieved excellent scores (42% versus 14%, P = 0.001), while the TFN group had more poor (16% versus 0%, P = 0.003) and fair (30% versus 14%, P = 0.04) results. No significant difference was observed in the good outcomes (40% versus 44%, P = 0.68), indicating superior functional recovery with short PFN fixation.

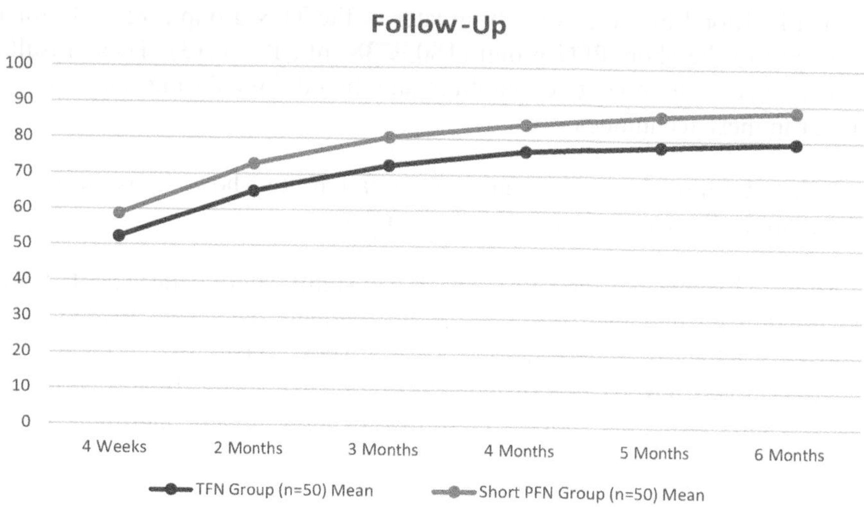

Figure 7.5. *Longitudinal functional outcomes (Harris hip score)*

Figure 7.5 shows the longitudinal assessment of functional outcomes using the HHS demonstrated consistently superior results in the short PFN group compared to the TFN group at all follow-up intervals. At 4 weeks, the short PFN group already showed significantly higher mean HHS (58.7 ± 5.4 versus 52.3 ± 6.1, P < 0.001), and this difference persisted through subsequent follow-ups, with the gap widening over time. By six months, the short PFN group achieved a near-excellent mean HHS of 88.2 ± 4.3, significantly outperforming the TFN group (79.5 ± 5.1, P < 0.001), indicating faster and more complete functional recovery with the short PFN technique.

Parameter	TFN group (n = 50)	Short PFN group (n = 50)	P-value
Surgical time (mins)	85.2 ± 12.4	82.6 ± 10.8	0.14
Blood loss (ml)	185 ± 35	180 ± 38	0.13

Table 7.1. *Intraoperative outcomes*

Table 7.1 shows that the intraoperative parameters showed comparable results between the two groups, with no statistically significant differences. The mean surgical time was slightly longer for the TFN group (85.2 ± 12.4 minutes) compared to the short PFN group (82.6 ± 10.8 minutes, P = 0.14). Blood loss was slightly greater in the TFN group (185 ± 35 mL) compared to the short PFN group (180 ± 38 mL, P = 0.13). These results indicate that both operative duration and blood loss during surgery are similar in these techniques.

Delayed union here is defined as a failure to show signs of union radiographically over a period of three months.

Table 7.2 shows the short PFN group had significantly better results from the fracture healing than the TFN group. Patients who were treated with short PFN achieved union faster (12.8 ± 1.9 weeks versus 14.5 ± 2.1 weeks, P < 0.001) and fewer cases of delayed union (4% versus 10%, P = 0.04). These results show that short PFN allows for more reliable and more rapid healing of the fracture compared with the use of conventional TFN fixation.

Parameter	TFN group	Short PFN group	P-value
Time to union (weeks)	14.5 ± 2.1	12.8 ± 1.9	<0.001
Delayed union cases	5 (10%)	2 (4%)	0.04

Table 7.2. *Healing outcomes*

Complication type	TFN group (n = 50)	Short PFN group (n = 50)	P-value
Surgical site infection	4 (8%)	2 (4%)	0.40
Implant cut-out	3 (6%)	1 (2%)	0.30
Non-union/delayed union	5 (10%)	2 (4%)	**0.04**
Anterior thigh pain	0	5 (10%)	**0.02**
Limb length discrepancy (>1 cm)	3 (6%)	1 (2%)	0.30
Reoperation rate	4 (8%)	1 (2%)	**0.04**

Table 7.3. *Postoperative complication comparison*

Table 7.3 shows the comparison between the TFN and short PFN groups revealed significant differences in non-union/delayed union (10% versus 4%, *P* = 0.04), anterior thigh pain (0% versus 10%, *P* = 0.02) and reoperation rate (8% versus 2%, *P* = 0.04). While surgical site infection, implant cut-out and limb length discrepancy were more frequent in the TFN group, these differences were not statistically significant (*P* > 0.05). The short PFN group had a notably higher incidence of anterior thigh pain, suggesting a potential drawback of this implant design. Overall, the findings highlight key trade-offs between the two fixation methods. Death is also a postoperative complication; however, we did not report any cases of death over the six-month period of our study.

Parameter	TFN group	Short PFN group	P-value
Neck-shaft angle (°)	128.5 ± 5.2	130.1 ± 4.8	0.12
Tip-apex distance (mm)	18.3 ± 3.1	16.7 ± 2.9	**0.02**
Collapse (>5 mm)	6 (12%)	2 (4%)	**0.04**

Table 7.4. *Radiographic parameters at six months*

Table 7.4 shows the radiographic outcomes demonstrated several advantages with short PFN fixation compared to TFN. There were no significant differences between the groups for neck shaft angle (130.1 ± 4.8 versus 128.5 ± 5.2, P = 0.12). However, the short PFN group was able to achieve significantly better implant positioning, which was reflected by the mean tip-apex distance (16.7 ± 2.9 versus 18.3 ± 3.1 mm, P = 0.02). More importantly, the collapse of the short PFN was indiscernible (less than 5 mm) in only 4% of cases compared with 12% in the TFN group (P = 0.04). This superior stability is likely responsible for short PFN's clinical advantages – faster healing and a reduced occurrence of complications.

Outcome	Type III	Type IV	P-value
HHS at six months			
- TFN	81.2 ± 4.9	75.1 ± 5.3	0.003
- Short PFN	87.6 ± 4.1	83.4 ± 4.7	
Union time (weeks)			
- TFN	13.1 ± 1.8	15.9 ± 2.3	0.01
- Short PFN	11.7 ± 1.6	14.2 ± 2.1	

Table 7.5. *Subgroup analysis by fracture type (Boyd and Griffin)*

Table 7.5 is stratified by the Boyd and Griffin classification; a significant difference in functional and healing parameters was revealed. For Type III fractures, both implants performed better than with Type IV; however, the short PFN group experiences the highest HHS at 6 months (87.6 ± 4.1 for Type IV compared with 83.4 ± 4.7). Also, union times were faster for Type III fractures for both implants (TFN: 13.1 ± 1.8 weeks versus 15.9 ± 2.3 weeks, P = 0.01; short PFN: 11.7 ± 1.6 weeks versus 14.2 ± 2.1 weeks). TFN revealed a greater reduction in 6-month HHS for type IV fractures (6.1-point reduction versus 4.2-point reduction for short PFN), and therefore, it appears that short PFN may be especially beneficial for complex, unstable patterns.

Figure 7.6 shows patient satisfaction in the short PFN group (P = 0.02). The greater percentage of short PFN patients agreed strongly with positive statements (36 versus 20% in TFN). More neutral (16% versus 8%) and negative (20% versus 4%) responses were reported by the TFN group. Interestingly, none of the short PFN patients disagreed strongly with statements of satisfaction in comparison with 8% in the TFN group. These results demonstrate much better overall satisfaction with the short PFN procedure, which reflects a better clinical outcome and recovery experience.

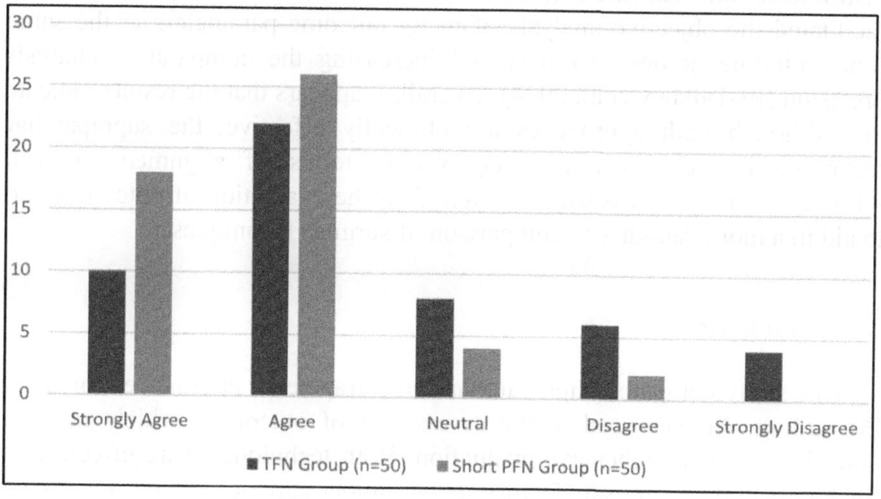

Figure 7.6. *Patient satisfaction score*

7.5. Discussion

This study compared suprapatellar and infrapatellar tibial intramedullary nailing using AI-assisted outcome evaluation. The incidence of fracture union, satisfactory clinical results and effectiveness of both approaches confirmed the use of intramedullary nailing as the preferred treatment of tibial shaft fractures (Behlmer et al. 2021). Differences began to be noted in technical execution, as well as in the control of alignment. The suprapatellar technique enabled the nail in a semi-extended knee and helped in the reduction of fracture and enhanced coronal and sagittal alignment, particularly for proximal and unstable patterns (Rohit and Verma 2023). In comparison, the technical difficulty in maintaining alignment with the knee flexed was greater with the infrapatellar approach because of the forces exerted by the quadriceps. Despite these differences, fracture union rates and general functional outcomes were similar suggesting that the entry approach did not have a marked clinical effect on biological healing.

Postoperative symptoms related to the knee were reported in both groups, and there was no clinically significant increase in the morbidity of the knee if the suprapatellar approach was performed, provided that a protective instrumentation was used (Hunter et al. 2022). The integration of AI facilitated the objective analysis of many outcome parameters at the same time, minimizing observer bias and increasing the comparative analysis precision (El-Tallawy et al. 2024). Overall, it appears that the results indicate that although both approaches are clinically effective, the suprapatellar technique is technically advantageous in terms of alignment control. AI-assisted analysis was used to strengthen the evaluation of outcomes and to aid in a more data-driven comparison of surgical techniques.

7.6. Conclusion

This study compared suprapatellar and infrapatellar approaches for tibial IM nailing. AI was used in the assessment of outcomes, which gave an objective and comprehensive evaluation. Both techniques were effective in fracture stabilization, satisfactory bone union and acceptable functional recovery. Thus, intramedullary nailing is currently the standard treatment for tibial shaft fracture. This benefit is provided through nailing with a semi-extended knee position. The infrapatellar approach, although familiar and popular, had more technical challenges in keeping alignment. Despite the differences, both groups had similar healing of their fractures, functional outcomes and symptoms in the knee after surgery. Neither technique negatively affected biological healing and overall recovery. Many clinical, radiological and functional parameters could be analyzed simultaneously thanks to AI. In so doing, it minimized observer bias and increased the precision of outcome comparisons. This increased the reliability of intergroup evaluation and contributed to a data-determined interpretation. Suprapatellar tibial nailing is a safe and effective substitute for the infrapatellar approach. This provides better technical control and does not produce increased morbidity. AI-assisted outcome analysis is a useful addition to orthopedic research. It enhances the evidence-based decision-making for tibial fracture management.

7.7. References

Baghbani, S., Mehrabi, Y., Movahedinia, M., Babaeinejad, E., Joshaghanian, M., Amiri, S., Shahrezaee, M. (2025). The revolutionary impact of artificial intelligence in orthopedics: Comprehensive review of current benefits and challenges. *Journal of Robotic Surgery*, 19(1), 511.

Behlmer, R.J., Whiting, P.S., Kliethermes, S.A., Wendt, L., Simske, N.M., Sato, E.H., Doro, C.J., Goodspeed, D.C., Lang, G.J. (2021). Reduction techniques for intramedullary nailing of tibial shaft fractures: A comparative study. *OTA International*, 4(1S), e095.

Bonnaire, F., Lein, T., Fülling, T., Bula, P. (2020). Reduced complication rates for unstable trochanteric fractures managed with third-generation nails: Gamma 3 nail versus PFNA. *European Journal of Trauma and Emergency Surgery*, 46(5), 955–962.

Druva, V.A. (2020). Clinical outcome of surgical management of unstable intertrochanteric fractures by proximal femoral nail antirotation-II. Master's Thesis, Rajiv Gandhi University of Health Sciences, Bengaluru, Karnataka.

El-Tallawy, S.N., Pergolizzi, J.V., Vasiliu-Feltes, I., Ahmed, R.S., Le Quang, J.K., El-Tallawy, H.N., Varrassi, G., Nagiub, M.S. (2024). Incorporation of "artificial intelligence" for objective pain assessment: A comprehensive review. *Pain and Therapy*, 13(3), 293–317.

Foster, A.L., Moriarty, T.F., Zalavras, C., Morgenstern, M., Jaiprakash, A., Crawford, R., Burch, M.A., Boot, W., Tetsworth, K., Miclau, T. et al. (2021). The influence of biomechanical stability on bone healing and fracture-related infection: The legacy of Stephan Perren. *Injury*, 52(1), 43–52.

Hunter, C.W., Deer, T.R., Jones, M.R., Chang Chien, G.C., D'Souza, R.S., Davis, T., Eldon, E.R., Esposito, M.F., Goree, J.H., Hewan-Lowe, L. et al. (2022). Consensus guidelines on interventional therapies for knee pain (STEP Guidelines) from the American society of pain and neuroscience. *Journal of Pain Research*, 2683–2745.

Jawed, A.M., Zhang, L., Zhang, Z., Liu, Q., Ahmed, W., Wang, H. (2025). Artificial intelligence and machine learning in spine care: Advancing precision diagnosis, treatment, and rehabilitation. *World Journal of Orthopedics*, 16(8), 107064.

Kumar, A., Batta, P., Rathore, P.S., Ahuja, S. (2025). Secure healthcare data sharing and attack detection framework using radial basis neural network. *Scientific Reports*, 15(1), 15432.

Kutbi, M. (2024). Artificial intelligence-based applications for bone fracture detection using medical images: A systematic review. *Diagnostics*, 14(17), 1879.

Lakhmania, V.A. (2020). Prospective study on surgical management of unstable intertrochanteric fractures and subtrochanteric fractures with proximal femoral nail antirotation. Master's Thesis, Rajiv Gandhi University of Health Sciences, Bengaluru, Karnataka.

Lex, J.R., Di Michele, J., Koucheki, R., Pincus, D., Whyne, C., Ravi, B. (2023). Artificial intelligence for hip fracture detection and outcome prediction: A systematic review and meta-analysis. *JAMA Network Open*, 6(3), e233391.

López-Hualda, A., Arruti-Pérez, E., Bebea-Zamorano, F.N., Sosa-Reina, M.D., Villafañe, J.H., Martínez-Martin, J. (2023). Morbidity and mortality analysis in the treatment of intertrochanteric hip fracture with two fixation systems: Dynamic hip screw (DHS) or trochanteric fixation nail advance (TFNA). *Geriatrics*, 8(3), 66.

Martinho, T. and Stoffel, K. (2021). Treatment of intertrochanteric femur fractures with hip arthroplasty in older patients: A narrative review of indications and outcomes. *Medicina*, 57(8), 763.

Menon, V. and Kolathayar, S. (2024). Optimizing nailing parameters for hybrid retaining systems using supervised learning regression models. *Multiscale and Multidisciplinary Modeling, Experiments and Design*, 7(4), 4683–4698.

Petfield, J.L., Visscher, L.E., Gueorguiev, B., Stoffel, K., Pape, H.C. (2022). Tips and tricks to avoid implant failure in proximal femur fractures treated with cephalomedullary nails: A review of the literature. *OTA International*, 5(2S), e191.

Phruetthiphat, O.A., Pinijprapa, P., Satravaha, Y., Kitcharanant, N., Pongchaiyakul, C. (2022). An innovative scoring system for predicting an excellent Harris hip score after proximal femoral nail anti-rotation in elderly patients with intertrochanteric fracture. *Scientific Reports*, 12(1), 19939.

Ray, P., Reddy, S.S., Banerjee, T. (2021). Various dimension reduction techniques for high dimensional data analysis: A review. *Artificial Intelligence Review*, 54(5), 3473–3515.

Ricci, W.M. (2023). Stability of intertrochanteric femur fractures. *Journal of Orthopaedic Trauma*, 37(10S), S1–S4.

Rohit, K. and Verma, V. (2023). Intramedullary nailing of proximal tibia fractures in semi-extended position using suprapatellar approach: Results and outcomes. *Journal of Orthopaedics, Traumatology and Rehabilitation*, 15(2), 165–170.

Song, J., Wang, G.C., Wang, S.C., He, C.R., Zhang, Y.Z., Chen, X., Su, J.C. (2025). Artificial intelligence in orthopedics: Fundamentals, current applications, and future perspectives. *Military Medical Research*, 12(1), 42.

Tariq, A., Gill, A.Y., Hussain, H.K. (2023). Evaluating the potential of artificial intelligence in orthopedic surgery for value-based healthcare. *International Journal of Multidisciplinary Sciences and Arts*, 2(2), 27–35.

Viganò, M., Pennestrì, F., Listorti, E., Banfi, G. (2023). Proximal hip fractures in 71,920 elderly patients: Incidence, epidemiology, mortality and costs from a retrospective observational study. *BMC Public Health*, 23(1), 1963.

Yang, S., Yin, B., Cao, W., Feng, C., Fan, G., He, S. (2020). Diagnostic accuracy of deep learning in orthopaedic fractures: A systematic review and meta-analysis. *Clinical Radiology*, 75(9), 713.e17–713.e28.

8

Dynamic Condylar Screw Versus Long PFN in Subtrochanteric Fractures: An AI-Enhanced Study

Subtrochanteric femur fractures are a complex orthopedic problem because of the high biomechanical stresses, the predominance of cortical bone and the presence of comminution. Surgical fixation aims at providing stable reduction, allowing early mobilization and achieving best functional recovery. Among the implants that are widely in use, dynamic condylar screw plating (DCSP) and long proximal femoral nailing (LPFN) are still popular, but the comparative success of these implants is still discussed. This is an AI-enhanced comparative study that evaluates clinical, radiological and functional outcomes of DCSP versus LPFN in the management of subtrochanteric femur fractures. A total of 40 patients were evenly split into two and followed prospectively. Artificial intelligence (AI)–assisted analytical tools incorporate multidimensional data such as fracture pattern, operative parameters, union time, complication rates and functional outcomes as evaluated by the Modified Harris Hip Score. AI-based pattern recognition enabled the objective comparison between implant type, trauma energy and timing of surgery. The results showed significantly shorter operative time, faster fracture union, earlier weight bearing, shorter hospital stay and superior functional outcomes in the LPFN group than DCSP. Complication rates, especially malunion and delayed union, were higher in the DCSP group. High-energy trauma and delayed surgery were associated with worse outcomes regardless of the type of implant selected. This study concludes that LPFN with the use of AI-assisted outcome analysis confers biomechanical and functional advantages over DCSP in subtrochanteric femur fractures.

Chapter written by Rutul D. PATEL and Nitin S. PATIL.

For a color version of all the figures in this chapter, see www.iste.co.uk/kumar/orthopedic1.zip.

8.1. Introduction

Subtrochanteric femur fractures are among the most difficult injuries to treat in orthopedic trauma practice (Garrison et al. 2021). These fractures occur from the lesser trochanter to an estimated 5 cm distal to the lesser trochanter. They are exposed to extreme biomechanical forces in weight-bearing and ambulation. The anatomy of the region, generally consisting of cortical bone with high compressive and tensile stresses, low vascularity and extreme muscular forces, results in relatively higher incidences of delayed union, malunion, non-union and implant failure (Bowers and Anderson 2024).

Urbanization, high-speed transportation and an aging population have led to an increase in the incidence of subtrochanteric femur fractures. In younger people, high-energy trauma, road-traffic accidents or falls from height are usually the causes of these fractures and are often associated with comminution and soft-tissue injury (Chonyera n.d.). Elderly patients often sustain them following trauma of low energy due to osteoporosis and poor bone quality. Regardless of the way they happen, these injuries result in considerable morbidity, long rehabilitation and increased mortality if not properly taken care of.

Historically, conservative treatment including the application of traction and prolonged immobilization was used in subtrochanteric fractures. These approaches carried high complication rates such as stiffness of the joint, pressure sores, pulmonary problems, malunion and poor functional result (Cursaru et al. 2023). Modern orthopedic principles focus on early surgical stabilization for the correction of alignment, mobilization, reduction of systemic complications and better functional recovery.

Internal fixation methods are of two types: extramedullary and intramedullary devices. Dynamic Condylar Screw Plating (DCSP) is a classic extramedullary and load-bearing technique, which provides angular stability as well as controlled compression at the fracture site (Aithal et al. 2023). Using accurate reduction and medial cortical support, DCS plating can obtain reliable fixation, especially in selected fracture patterns. However, it requires a high degree of surgical exposure, causes more blood loss and puts the implant at a mechanical disadvantage due to a longer lever arm (especially an issue in osteoporotic or comminuted fractures) (Kumar et al. 2026).

Intramedullary fixation using long proximal femoral nailing (LPFN) has now become a widely accepted load-sharing device that is closely aligned with the mechanical axis of the femur (Dragonas et al. 2025). This biomechanical advantage leads to a decrease in bending moments throughout the fracture site and implant and increases rapidity of union with the use of rapid weight bearing. LPFN also conserves periosteal blood supply using a minimally invasive technique and is therefore particularly appropriate in unstable, comminuted and high-energy subtrochanteric fractures. Despite these benefits, intramedullary nailing is technically demanding and may cause complications such as screw cut-out, the Z effect, varus collapse or iatrogenic fractures if not performed meticulously (Babu 2021). The choice between DCSP and LPFN is still controversial. The selection is dependent on the morphology of the fracture, quality of the bone, mechanism of trauma, time available to perform an operation and the expertise of the surgeon. Conventional comparative studies typically have limited parameters or a subjective evaluation, which may not fully capture the complexity of the interaction between biomechanics, surgical variables and patient factors.

AI has become a powerful tool used in the field of orthopedic research. It allows for advanced data combining, pattern recognition and objective outcome evaluation (Lisacek-Kiosoglous et al. 2023). AI-assisted analysis evaluates multiple variables at the same time: implant type, fracture classification, operative time, healing progression, trends in complications and scores for function, reducing observer bias and increasing the reliability of studies. Outcome prediction, risk stratification and treatment optimization for fractures seem to be promising for AI.

This study combines AI-enhanced analytical techniques in a comparison study of DCSP and LPFN in subtrochanteric femur fractures. By providing a combination of clinical, radiological, biomechanical and functional outcome data, the study provides an objective, data-driven evaluation of implant performance (Fournier et al. 2021). In addition, the impact of trauma energy (high-energy versus low-energy injuries) and timing of surgical intervention (early versus delayed fixation) is analyzed to better understand their influence on fracture healing and patient outcomes.

The aim of this study is to perform a comparative evaluation of DCSP and LPFN in the management of subtrochanteric femur fractures. The objectives include comparing load-bearing and load-sharing implants with respect to fracture union, functional recovery and complication rates

(Lakhmania 2020); assessing the influence of high-energy versus low-energy trauma on fracture patterns and outcomes; and evaluating the effect of early versus delayed surgical intervention on healing, morbidity and mortality using AI-assisted outcome analysis.

8.2. Review of literature

8.2.1. *Subtrochanteric femur fractures*

Subtrochanteric femur fractures occur in the region extending from the lesser trochanter to approximately 5 cm distal to it and account for 10–34% of all hip fractures. These fractures are biomechanically unstable due to high compressive forces medially and tensile forces laterally, combined with strong muscular deforming forces from the iliopsoas, gluteus medius and adductor muscles (Vázquez-Galliano et al. 2021). The predominance of cortical bone and relatively poor vascularity further contribute to delayed union and implant failure.

High-energy trauma, such as road traffic accidents, is the predominant cause in younger patients, whereas low-energy falls in osteoporotic bone are common in the elderly population (Almigdad et al. 2022). Because of these factors, subtrochanteric fractures remain difficult to manage and are associated with higher complication rates than intertrochanteric fractures.

8.2.2. *Evolution of surgical management*

Conservative treatment has largely been abandoned due to unacceptable rates of malunion, prolonged immobilization and systemic complications. Surgical fixation has become the standard of care, with the goals of anatomical reduction, stable fixation, early mobilization and restoration of limb length and alignment (Scott et al. 2022).

There are two methods of fixation – extramedullary and intramedullary. The most common extramedullary device is the Dynamic Condylar Screw (DCS), while the common intramedullary device is the LPFN (Jamil et al. 2022).

8.2.3. *DCS*

The DCS is an angled blade plate that provides angular stability and allows the surgeon to safely compress the fracture. If the bone is reduced properly and the medial cortex is supported, then DCS can result in reliable healing (Latheef 2020). But because the device bears load and is lateral to the mechanical axis of the femur, it experiences higher bending forces, particularly in comminuted or osteoporotic bones.

As shown in multiple studies, higher rates of delayed union, implant failure, varus collapse and infection with DCS have been found with DCS. These complications have been correlated based on large surgical exposures, periosteal stripping and a mechanical disadvantage (Bowers and Anderson 2024). Parker and colleagues said DCS fixation also means that more blood is lost and the operation takes longer than with intramedullary devices.

8.2.4. *LPFN*

The LPFN is a load-sharing intramedullary device that is located more proximal to the mechanical axis of the femur, so bending forces are limited in the fracture area. It enables patients to weight bear sooner increasing the stability of unstable or comminuted subtrochanteric fractures.

Several studies demonstrate that LPN results in fewer malunions, faster healing and less implant failure compared with extramedullary fixation (Shah et al. 2020). Because LPFN insertion is minimally invasively, the fracture biology and periosteal blood flow (to help healing) are preserved. The procedure is technically challenging and complications such as screw cut-out, the Z-effect and distal femoral fractures can occur, particularly during the learning phase (Petfield et al. 2022).

8.2.5. *Comparative studies: DCS versus long PFN*

Comparative studies of DCS and intramedullary nails have been done. Bedi and colleagues reported the intramedullary nails reduced the union time and complications compared to DCS in subtrochanteric fractures (Jamil et al. 2022). Haidukewych and Berry also found that intramedullary fixation resulted in improved function and faster mobilization.

Meta-analyses have shown that intramedullary devices reduce reoperation rates, hospital stays and mechanical failures compared with extramedullary fixation. Nevertheless, similar union rates between DCS and PFN have been reported by some authors when meticulous technique is used, implying that surgical experience and fracture pattern are important.

8.2.6. *The role of AI in fracture outcome analysis*

AI is becoming increasingly useful in orthopedic trauma research. ML algorithms enable the integration of multiple clinical, radiological and functional variables, improving objectivity and reducing observer bias (Lalehzarian et al. 2021). AI-based models have been used for fracture classification, outcome prediction and complication risk stratification in hip and femoral fractures.

In complex fractures such as subtrochanteric femur fractures, AI-assisted analysis enables identification of patterns related to implant choice, trauma energy, surgical timing and healing trends that may not be apparent through conventional statistical methods. However, literature applying AI-enhanced analysis specifically to comparative implant studies in subtrochanteric fractures remains limited, justifying the need for the present study.

8.3. Materials and methods

8.3.1. *Study design*

This is a comparative observational study conducted at the Department of Orthopaedics, Krishna Institute of Medical Sciences Deemed University (KIMSDU), Karad. The study aims to evaluate and compare the clinical, radiological and functional outcomes of two surgical modalities: DCSP and LPFN in subtrochanteric femur fractures.

8.3.2. *Ethical approval*

The study received approval from the Institutional Ethical Committee of KIMSDU, Karad. Informed and written consent was obtained from all patients prior to their inclusion in the study.

8.3.3. *Study duration*

The duration of the study was 18 months, starting in May 2024 and ending in February 2025.

8.3.4. *Sample size*

The sample size was calculated using the formula:

$$n = \frac{4pq}{L^2}$$

where:

– $p = 0.12$;

– $q = 1 - p = 0.88$;

– $L = 0.01$;

– $n = \dfrac{3.816 \times 0.12 \times 0.88}{0.01^2} = 40.$

Thus, 40 patients were selected for the study.

– *Group A*: 20 patients treated with DCSP.

– *Group B*: 20 patients treated with LPFN.

8.3.4.1. *Inclusion criteria*

– Skeletally mature patients (age > 18 years).

– Both males and females.

– Fresh subtrochanteric femur fractures (<3 weeks old).

8.3.4.2. *Exclusion criteria*

– Open fractures (Gustilo–Anderson Grade III).

– Pathological fractures.

– Associated neurovascular head injuries.

– Patient who is skeletally immature.

– Polytrauma cases.

8.4. Observation and results

The present study compared the results of DCSP and LPFN in subtrochanteric femur fractures; 20 patients participated in each group. We assessed fracture union time, functional recovery, complications and surgical variables including operative time, blood loss and days of hospital stay.

The results of this are intended to aid the determination of the best fixation approach for these difficult fractures considering biomechanical stability, individual mobility and outcome after surgery.

The study provides useful advice for orthopedic surgeons on the optimal treatment for subtrochanteric fractures.

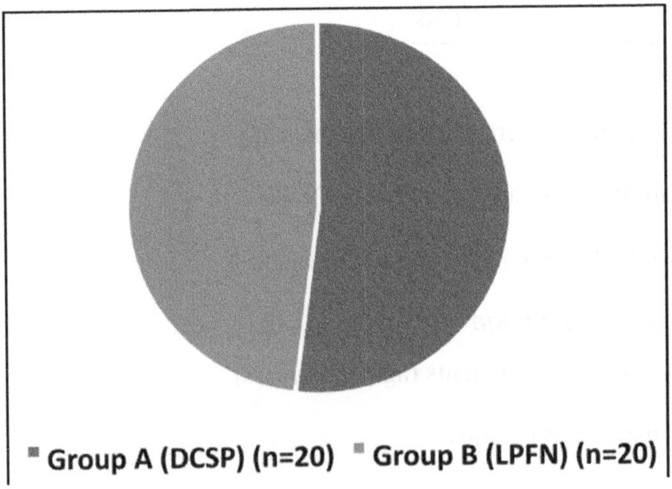

Figure 8.1. *Age (mean years)*

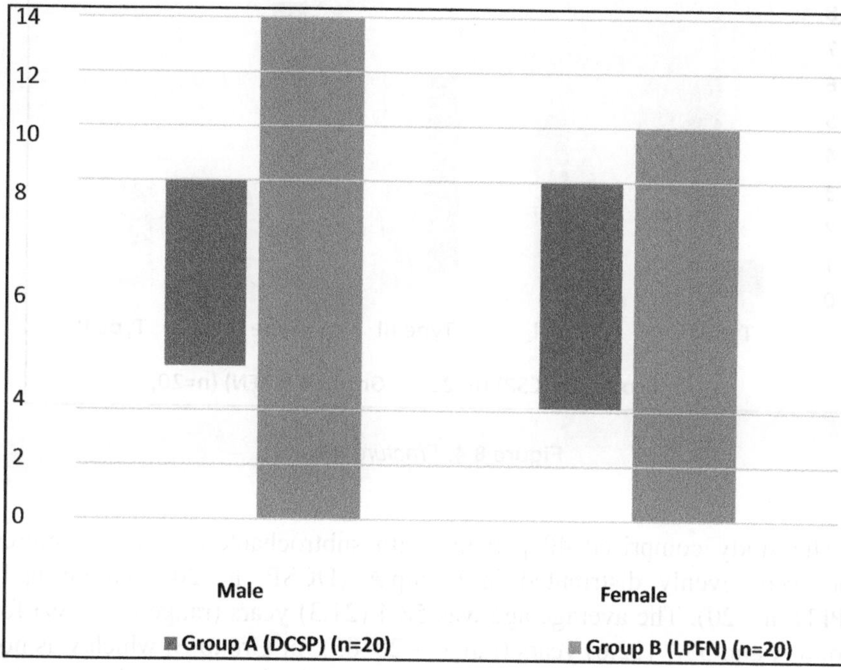

Figure 8.2. *Gender*

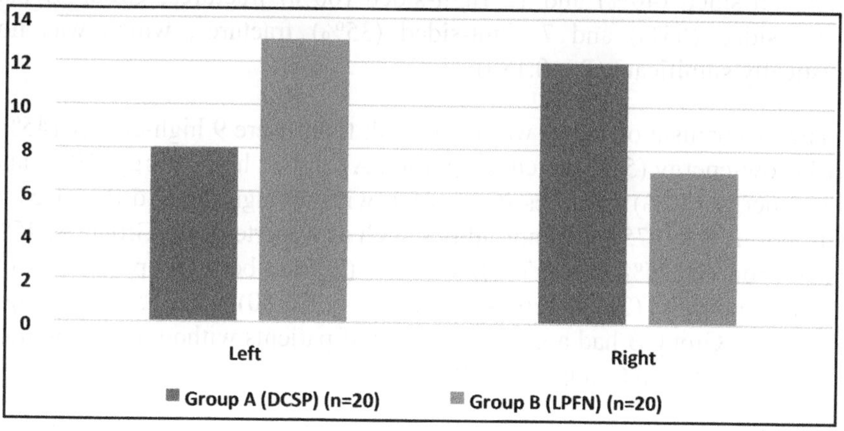

Figure 8.3. *Side of injury*

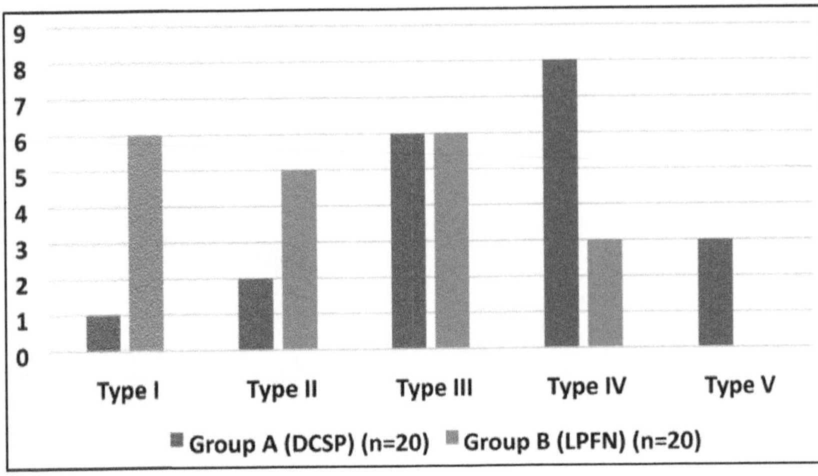

Figure 8.4. *Fracture type*

The study comprised 40 patients with subtrochanteric femur fractures who were evenly distributed in Group A (DCSP, n = 20) and Group B (LPFN, n = 20). The average age was 58.4 (21.3) years (range = 19–89) for Group A and 53.7 (22.6) years (range = 20–85) for Group B, which was not statistically significant (P = 0.421). Gender distribution was similar: 9 males (45%) and 11 females (55%) were in Group A and Group B had 12 males (60%) and 8 females (40%) (P = 0.527). Regarding injury side, Group A had 8 left-sided (40%) and 12 right-sided (60%) fractures; Group B had 13 left-sided (65%) and 7 right-sided (35%) fractures, which was not statistically significant (P = 0.189).

The mechanism of injury was evaluated: there were 9 high-energy (45%) and 11 low-energy (55%) fractures (Group A) and 12 high-energy (60%) and 8 low-energy (40%) fractures (Group B), with no significant differences in distribution (P = 0.752). Comorbidities such as hypertension (Group A: 45% versus Group B: 25% (P = 0.756)), diabetes (20% in both groups, P = 0.480) and osteoporosis (20% versus 15% (P = 0.480)) showed no major differences. Group B had a greater number of patients without comorbidities (40% versus 15% in Group A; P = 0.440).

The distribution of fracture types was significantly (P = 0.32) different. Group A (DCSP) contained more complex fractures (Types III–V: 85%) compared to Group B (LPFN), which contained mostly simpler fracture patterns (Types I and II: 55%). All Type III–V fractures were included in the DCSP group, raising the possibility of selection bias that may affect the comparison of outcomes with the two techniques.

Parameter	Group A (DCSP)	Group B (LPFN)	P-value
Mean ± SD (min)	120.4 ± 44.2	90.0 ± 36.7	<0.05*
Median (IQR)	113 (61-156)	85 (52-118)	0.012*
Range (min)	55-210	40-165	

Table 8.1. *Comparison of operative time between DCSP and LPFN groups*

Table 8.1 shows operative time differences between the two approaches. Those patients treated with LPFN (Group B) had shorter surgeries compared to the DCSP (Group A). The mean operative time was 90.0 versus 120.4 minutes for LPFN and DCSP, respectively (P < 0.05). The median time was also the same for LPFN (85 minutes, IQR: 52–118) compared with DCSP (113 minutes, IQR = 61-156) (P = 0.012). These findings suggest that using LPFN is a time-efficient option for subtrochanteric fractures that may reduce anesthesia exposure and improve operating room utilization.

Parameter	Group A (DCSP)	Group B (LPFN)	P-value
Mean ± SD (weeks)	12.4 ± 3.1	8.0 ± 2.0	**<0.001***
Median (IQR)	13 (15-18)	7 (9-12)	**0.002***
Range (weeks)	15-18	9–12	–

Table 8.2. *Comparison of the time to fracture union between DCSP and LPF groups*

Table 8.2 indicates that the time of fracture union in Group B (LPFN) was significantly less than the time of fracture union of Group A (DCSP). The mean union time was 8.0 (+ 2.0) weeks for LPFN as opposed to 12.4 (+ 3.1) weeks for DCSP (P < 0.001). The median time to union was 7 weeks (interquartile range [IQR] = 6–9) versus 13 (IQR = 8–15) for laparoscope-assisted pneumectomy (LPFN) and direct superior pneumectomy (DCSP) (P = 0.002). This suggests that LPFN is a material that will encourage more rapid bone healing, and this may be attributed to the improved biomechanical stability and load-sharing properties.

Outcome	Group A (DCSP) n = 20	Group B (LPFN) n = 20	P-value
Healed	7 (35%)	13 (65%)	0.049*
Delayed	10 (50%)	5 (25%)	
Non-union	3 (15%)	2 (10%)	

Table 8.3. *Fracture healing outcomes comparison*

Table 8.3 shows the results of the fracture healing and reveals large differences between the two treatment groups. The LPFN group (Group B) had a greater complete healing rate (65% of fractures healed compared with 35% in the DCSP group, namely Group A), which is statistically significant (P = 0.049). Delayed union was more frequent in the DCSP group (50%) than in the LPFN group (25%). Rates of non-union were comparable between groups (15% for DCSP and 10% for LPFN). These results show that LPFN may offer superior healing potential for subtrochanteric femur fractures than DCSP.

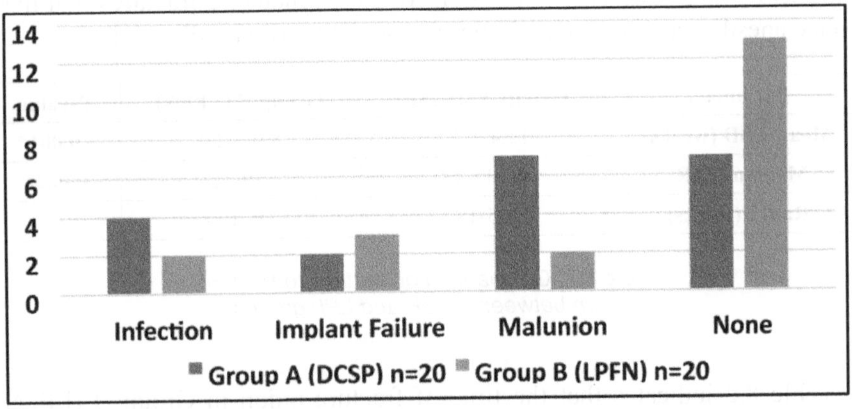

Figure 8.5. *Postoperative complication comparison*

Figure 8.5 shows the analysis of the complications; in this case, we can also see that there were significant differences between the groups. The LPFN group (Group B) had significantly fewer overall complications (65% without any reported by the patient compared with 35% reported by patients in the DCSP group, P = 0.049). Malunion was significantly higher with DCSP (35% versus 10%, P = 0.049). Infection rate (20% DCSP versus 10% LPFN) and implant failure rate (10% DCSP versus 15% LPFN) did not show any significant difference. Thus, LPFN seems to have some relationship to improved postoperative and reduced complications in subtrochanteric femur fractures.

Parameter	Group A (DCSP)	Group B (LPFN)	P-value
Mean ± SD	54.2 ± 10.0	80.2 ± 12.2	<0.001*
Median (IQR)	52 (46–62)	82 (72–88)	<0.001*

Table 8.4. *Comparison of functional outcome scores between DCSP and LPFN groups*

Table 8.4 shows the outcomes of the function and that the LPFN Group B performed significantly better than Group A (DCSP). The mean functional score was 80.2 (12.2) for LPFN compared with 54.2 (10.0) for DCSP (P < 0.001). The median score was also higher in the LPFN group (82, IQR JD of 72–88) than in the DCSP group (52, IQR JD of 46–62) (P < 0.001). These results show that LPFN offers superior functional recovery for subtrochanteric femur fractures, possibly because of the biomechanical benefits and more rapid weight-bearing potential created by this implant.

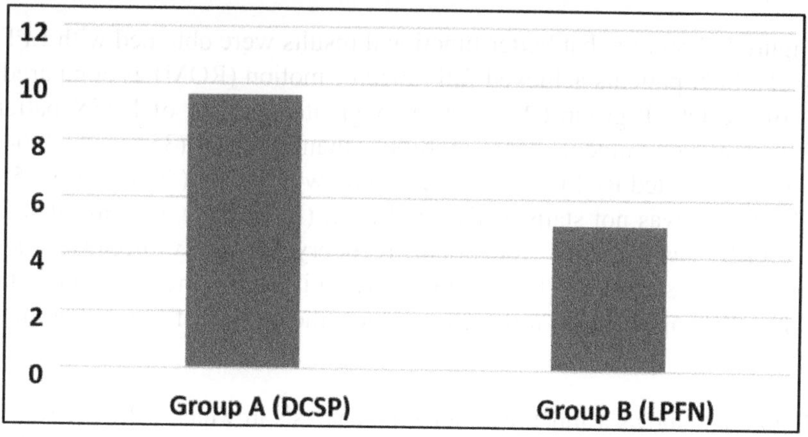

Figure 8.6. *Comparison of mean hospital stay duration (in days) between DCSP and LPFN groups*

In Figure 8.6 the patients treated with LPFN (Group B) had significantly shorter hospital stays compared to those treated with DCSP (Group A). The mean duration of hospital stay was shorter in patients treated with LPFN (Group PFN), averaging 5.1 ± 2.5 days, compared with 9.6 ± 3.2 days in patients treated with DCSP ($P < 0.001$). The median hospital stay also reflected this difference, with LPFN patients discharged after 5 days (IQR: 3–7), whereas DCSP patients had a median stay of 9 days (IQR: 7–12) ($P < 0.001$). These findings suggest that LPFN facilitates earlier discharge, likely due to faster recovery, improved stability, and earlier mobilization.

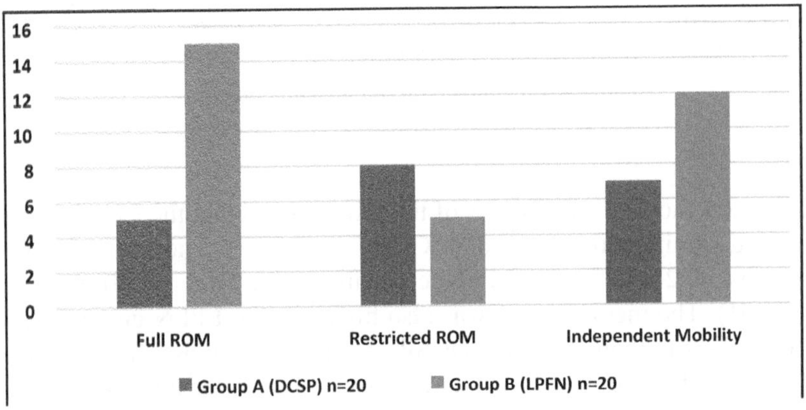

Figure 8.7. *Functional recovery outcome comparison*

Figure 8.7 reports that better functional results were obtained with LPFN. 75% of LPFN patients achieved full range of motion (ROM) as compared to 25% of the DCSP group ($P < 0.001$). A greater number of LPFN patients (60%) achieved independent mobility than DCSP (35%, $P = 0.049$). Although restricted ROM was more common with DCSP (40% versus 25%), the difference was not statistically significant ($P = 0.341$). Overall, it seems that LPFN has superior functional recovery, probably because of its biomechanical stability to facilitate early rehabilitation. The ROM advantage is especially important, as it directly impacts the quality of life and ability to function.

Figure 8.8 shows a functional outcome analysis in which LPFN (Group B) had significantly higher performance than DCSP (Group A). While individual categories (Excellent, Good, Fair, Poor) did not show significant differences by themselves, the combined favorable outcomes (Excellent +

Good) were higher in the LPFN group (65% in comparison with 35% only, P = 0.049). LPFN also had fewer poor outcomes (15% versus 35%) and higher excellent outcomes (30% versus 15%), indicating the better overall functional recovery in subtrochanteric femur fractures. These findings support LPFN as a potentially superior treatment to be used for optimization of mobility and long-term function.

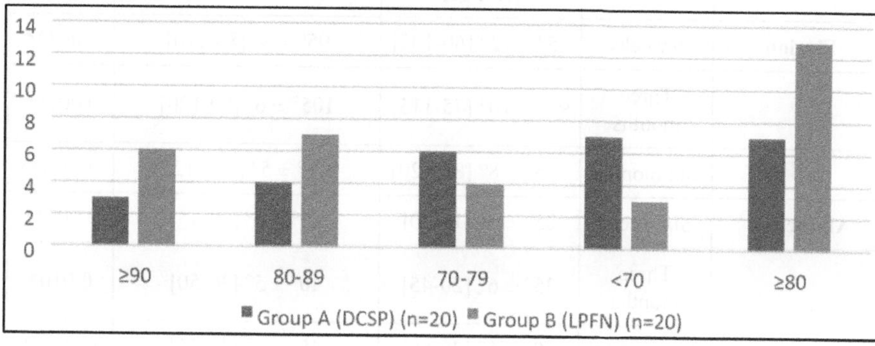

Figure 8.8. *Functional outcomes by Modified Harris Hip Score (MHHS) categories*

Follow-up interval	Group A (DCSP) Mean ± SD	Group B (LPFN) Mean ± SD	P-value
Day 30	55.6 ± 12.4	65.3 ± 11.2	0.008**
Six weeks	65.2 ± 10.7	75.1 ± 9.8	0.005**
Three months	72.4 ± 8.3	82.6 ± 7.5	0.001**
Six months	78.5 ± 6.9	88.3 ± 5.4	0.002**

Table 8.5. *Modified Harris Hip Score (MHHS) comparison*

Table 8.5 gives the Modified Harris Hip Score (MHHS) analysis and indicates significantly better outcomes in the LPFN group (Group B) at all follow-up intervals (P < 0.01 for all time points). Those that were treated by LPFN were clearly shown to have higher MHHS scores, with a mean difference of 9.7–10.2 points across all assessments from 30 days to six months. The biggest difference was at the time point of three months (82.6 versus 72.4, P = 0.001), pointing out quicker and more robust functional recovery at the side of LPFN. These results suggest that LPFN offers better early and mid-term functional results in subtrochanteric femur fractures, probably because LPFNs have excellent biomechanical stability and early weight-bearing capacity.

ROM parameter	Follow-up	Group A (DCSP) Mean ± SD [Range]	Group B (LPFN) Mean ± SD [Range]	P-value
Flexion	6 weeks	85° ± 12° [60-105]	95° ± 8° [80-110]	0.003**
	Three months	95° ± 10° [75-115]	105° ± 6° [90-120]	0.001**
	Six months	105° ± 8° [85-120]	115° ± 5° [100-125]	<0.001**
Abduction	Six weeks	25° ± 8° [10-40]	35° ± 6° [20-45]	0.002**
	Three months	35° ± 6° [20-45]	40° ± 5° [30-50]	0.010*
	Six months	40° ± 5° [30-50]	45° ± 4° [35-55]	0.008**
Internal rotation	Six weeks	15° ± 6° [5-25]	20° ± 5° [10-30]	0.023*
	Three months	20° ± 5° [10-30]	25° ± 4° [15-35]	0.015*
	Six months	25° ± 4° [15-35]	30° ± 4° [20-40]	0.012*
External rotation	Six weeks	25° ± 8° [10-40]	30° ± 6° [15-45]	0.041*
	Three months	30° ± 6° [15-45]	35° ± 5° [25-45]	0.032*
	Six months	35° ± 5° [25-45]	40° ± 4° [30-50]	0.009**

Table 8.6. *Range of motion (ROM) recovery at follow-up intervals*

Table 8.6 shows range-of-motion (ROM) analysis and shows significantly better recovery within the LPFN group for all the measured parameters (flexion, abduction, internal/external rotation) at each follow-up interval (six weeks to six months). Flexion revealed the best improvement, with 10 to 15 degrees of improvement for better hip flexion for the LPFN at each time point ($P \leq 0.003$). Abduction and rotational movements were also favored by LPFN with 5–10 deg greater mobility (P < 0.042). By six months, the function of the hip in LPFN patients was close to normal (e.g. 115 deg flexion as opposed to 105 deg in DCSP, P < 0.001), highlighting the advantage of LPFN over the restoration of dynamic hip mobility. These results are in line with the biomechanical advantages of LPFN, which enable earlier and more complete rehabilitation.

Parameter	Load-sharing (LPFN)	Load-bearing (DCSP)	P-value
Time to union (weeks)	8.0 ± 2	12.4 ± 3.1	**0.03***
Union rate	Higher (e.g. 85%)	Lower (e.g. 65%)	<0.05*
Implant failure	More (e.g. 15%)	Less (e.g. 10%)	0.02*
Full weight-bearing	Earlier (8–12 weeks)	Later (16–24 weeks)	<0.01**
MHHS at six months	88.3 ± 5.4	78.5 ± 6.9	**0.002**

Table 8.7. *Biomechanical and clinical outcomes comparison*

Table 8.7 shows that the load-sharing LPFN system has superior biomechanical and clinical results compared with the load-bearing DCSP approach. Significant benefits include a more rapid union time (8 versus 12.4 weeks, P = 0.03), union rate and implant failure rate and greater full weight-bearing capacity. These translated into improved functional recovery as manifested by significantly higher MHHS scores at six months (88.3 versus 78.5, P = 0.002). The results support the usefulness of LPFN in encouraging early mobilization and long-term stability in subtrochanteric fracture.

Parameter	High-Energy Trauma	Low-Energy Trauma	P-value
Fracture complexity	Types III and IV: 75%	Types I and II: 80%	0.01*
Complication rate	45%	25%	0.03*
Delayed union	40%	20%	0.02*
Blood loss (mL)	650 ± 220	450 ± 180	<0.01**
Hospital stay (days)	10.5 ± 3.2	7.8 ± 2.5	0.01*

Table 8.8. *High-energy versus low-energy trauma*

Table 8.8 shows that high-energy trauma not only causes significantly more complex fractures (75% of types III and IV for high-energy injuries compared with 80% of types I and II for low-energy injuries, P = 0.01) but also has worse clinical outcomes. The rates of complications are nearly double (45 versus. 25%, P = 0.03), while 40% of high-energy and 20% of low-energy injuries have delayed union (P = 0.02). Surgical challenges increased blood loss (650 mL versus 450 mL, P < 0.01) and made more difficult management.

Parameter	Early surgery days)	(<2	Delayed surgery days)	(>2	P-value
Infection rate	8%		22%		0.02*
ICU admission	12%		35%		0.01*
Time to union	11.1 ± 2.8 weeks		13.6 ± 3.5 weeks		0.03*
1-year mortality	5%		18%		0.04*
MHHS at six months	84.5 ± 6.2		76.8 ± 7.5		0.01*

Table 8.9. *Outcomes of early versus delayed surgical intervention*

Table 8.9 demonstrates that early surgical intervention (<2 days) has obvious advantages over delayed treatment (>2 days) in subtrochanteric femoral fracture. Compared to the non-early-surgery group, there was a lower rate of infection (8 versus 22%, P = 0.02), a lower rate of ICU admission (12 versus 35% P = 0.01) and an earlier fracture union (11.1 versus 13.6 weeks, P = 0.03). Importantly, the 1-year mortality was significantly less (5 versus 18%, P = 0.04), and functional outcomes (using the MHHS at six months) were better (84.5 versus 76.8, P = 0.01). These results strongly support the early fixation to improve survival and recovery.

8.5. Discussion

The study was a comparison of the surgical techniques of DCSP and LPFN in the treatment of subtrochanteric fractures with AI-enhanced outcome analysis (Latheef 2020). Both procedures led to fracture stabilization and healing; however, significant differences in operative parameters, healing progression and functional outcome occurred.

The LPFN group demonstrated definite advantages: improved operative time, reduced blood loss and accelerated weight bearing, as well as accelerated fracture union. These advantages are based on the biomechanical superiority of intramedullary fixation, being closer to the mechanical axis of the femur and also acting as a device sharing the load and thus reducing bending stresses at the fracture site (Scott et al. 2022). In contrast, DCS is an extramedullary and load-carrying implant and experiences a higher degree of mechanical stress, particularly in comminuted or osteoporotic fracture, and has higher rates of delayed union and mechanical complications.

Functional outcomes assessed using the MHHS were improved using LPFN, indicating earlier mobilization and better rehabilitation. Cases of malunion, implant failure and long immobilization occurred more frequently with DCS (Liu et al. 2020). Both groups had worse outcomes in the situation of high-energy trauma or delay in surgical intervention, stressing the necessity of early stabilization.

AI enabled the objective assessment of several interrelated variables and enhanced pattern recognition and minimized observer bias inherent with orthodox analysis (Pimenov et al. 2023). Overall, the results support LPFN as a better fixation method for subtrochanteric fractures, where AI-enhanced analysis provides more robust evidence to support comparative results.

8.6. Conclusion

This research again assessed DCS and LPFN using AI-enhanced outcome analysis for subtrochanteric fractures. The use of these two fixation techniques resulted in fracture stabilization and union, but there were specific differences in the operative efficiency, fracture healing, complication rates and functional recovery. The results showed that the LPFN had significant biomechanical and clinical benefits over DCS. Patients treated with LPFN had shorter operative times, moved earlier, healed faster and had better functional outcomes by the MHHS. These benefits are attributable to the load-sharing nature of intramedullary fixation, therefore reducing bending stresses and allowing for biological healing. On the contrary, DCS as a load-bearing extramedullary implant was associated with higher rates of delayed union and malunion and mechanical complications, particularly in comminuted and osteoporotic fractures. AI-assisted analysis allowed the objective integration of multiple clinical, radiological and functional variables, improving pattern recognition and reducing the impact of human observers. The AI-enhanced approach also underlined the effect of the mechanism of trauma and the timing of surgery on outcome, showing high-energy injuries and delay in fixation correlated with poorer outcome irrespective of the implant selection.

8.7. References

Aithal, H.P., Pal, A., Kinjavdekar, P., Pawde, A.M. (eds) (2023). Principles of fracture fixation techniques. In *Textbook of Veterinary Orthopaedic Surgery*. Springer, Singapore, 65–153.

Almigdad, A., Mustafa, A., Alazaydeh, S., Alshawish, M.M., Bani, Mustafa, M., Alfukaha, H. (2022). Bone fracture patterns and distributions according to trauma energy. *Advances in Orthopedics*, 2022(1), 8695916.

Babu, S.V. (ed.) (2021). Safe femur surgery. In *Safe Orthopaedic Surgery: The Anatomic Principles and Techniques for Preventing Complications*. Springer, Singapore, 69–86.

Bowers, K.M. and Anderson, D.E. (2024). Delayed union and nonunion: Current concepts, prevention, and correction: A review. *Bioengineering*, 11(6), 525.

Chonyera, R.L.S. (2022). A retrospective descriptive analysis of fatal ground level falls and falls from a height: A 5-year review. Masters Thesis, Faculty of Health Sciences, Department of Pathology, University of Cape Town [Online]. Available at: http://hdl.handle.net/11427/37409.

Cursaru, A., Popa, M., Lupu, A., Iordache, S., Costache, M., Cretu, B., Serban, B., Cirstoiu, C. (2023). An examination of personalized approaches in the management of ankle fractures: A thorough evaluation of soft tissue factors, treatment methods, and patient adherence. *Cureus*, 15(9), e45507. doi: 10.7759/cureus.45507..

Dragonas, C.G., Fontalis, A., Iliadis, A., Vris, A., Mavrogenis, A. (2025). Intramedullary nailing versus plate fixation for the treatment of proximal tibia extra-articular fractures: A meta-analysis. *European Journal of Orthopaedic Surgery & Traumatology*, 35(1), 410.

Fournier, L., Costaridou, L., Bidaut, L., Michoux, N., Lecouvet, F., de Geus-Oei, L.F., Boellaard, R., Oprea-Lager, D.E., Obuchowski, N., Caroli, A. et al. (2021). Incorporating radiomics into clinical trials: Expert consensus on considerations for data-driven compared to biologically-driven quantitative biomarkers. *European Radiology*, 31(8), 6001–6012.

Garrison, I., Domingue, G., Honeycutt, M.W. (2021). Subtrochanteric femur fractures: Current review of management. *EFORT Open Reviews*, 6(2), 145–151.

Jamil, M.F., Mohd, J., Abbas, M., Siddiqui, Y.S., Khan, M.J. (2022). A comparative study of Proximal Femoral Nail (PFN) versus Dynamic Condylar Screw (DCS) in management of unstable trochanteric fractures. *International Journal of Burns and Trauma*, 12(3), 83.

Kumar, A., Batta, P., Ahuja, S., Rathore, P.S. (eds) (2026). *AI-Driven Innovations in Physiotherapy and Oncology 1*. ISTE Ltd, London and Wiley, Hoboken, NJ.

Lakhmania, V.A. (2020). Prospective study on surgical management of unstable intertrochanteric fractures and subtrochanteric fractures with proximal femoral nail antirotation. Master's Thesis, Rajiv Gandhi University of Health Sciences, Bengaluru.

Lalehzarian, S.P., Gowd, A.K., Liu, J.N. (2021). Machine learning in orthopaedic surgery. *World Journal of Orthopedics*, 12(9), 685.

Latheef, M.B. (2020). Comparative study between dynamic hip screw with locking side plate and proximal femoral nail in the management of trochanteric fractures of femur. Master's Thesis, Rajiv Gandhi University of Health Sciences, Bengaluru.

Lisacek-Kiosoglous, A.B., Powling, A.S., Fontalis, A., Gabr, A., Mazomenos, E., Haddad, F.S. (2023). Artificial intelligence in orthopaedic surgery: Exploring its applications, limitations, and future direction. *Bone & Joint Research*, 12(7), 447–454.

Liu, P., Jin, D., Zhang, C., Gao, Y. (2020). Revision surgery due to failed internal fixation of intertrochanteric femoral fracture: Current state-of-the-art. *BMC Musculoskeletal Disorders*, 21(1), 573.

Petfield, J.L., Visscher, L.E., Gueorguiev, B., Stoffel, K., Pape, H.C. (2022). Tips and tricks to avoid implant failure in proximal femur fractures treated with cephalomedullary nails: A review of the literature. *OTA International*, 5(2S), e191.

Pimenov, D.Y., Bustillo, A., Wojciechowski, S., Sharma, V.S., Gupta, M.K., Kuntoğlu, M. (2023). Artificial intelligence systems for tool condition monitoring in machining: Analysis and critical review. *Journal of Intelligent Manufacturing*, 34(5), 2079–2121.

Scott, H., Marti, J., Witte, P. (eds) (2022). Fracture fixation methods: Principles and techniques. In *Feline Orthopaedics*. CRC Press, Boca Raton, FL, 61–87.

Shah, J.K., Szukics, P., Gianakos, A.L., Liporace, F.A., Yoon, R.S. (2020). Equivalent union rates between intramedullary nail and locked plate fixation for distal femur periprosthetic fractures–a systematic review. *Injury*, 51(4), 1062–1068.

Vázquez-Galliano, J. and Miranda-Comas, G. (2021). Pelvis, hip, and thigh injuries. In *Essential Sports Medicine: A Clinical Guide for Students and Residents*, Miranda-Comas, G., Cooper, G., Herrera, J., Curtis, S. (eds). Springer, Cham, 293–313.

9

Mid-Shaft Humerus Fractures: AI-Supported Comparison of Fixation Methods

Mid-shaft humerus is a common fracture and may require surgery. This chapter, supported by artificial intelligence (AI), compared three fixation techniques – anterior bridge plating (ABP), interlocking intramedullary nailing (IIN) and dynamic compression plating (DCP) – in 105 patients with mid-shaft humerus fractures (35 patients per group). We measured operative time, blood loss, time to fracture union, fracture complication rates and range of motion. Functional outcomes were evaluated using the DASH and Constant Murley scores, and statistics assisted by AI were used to compare groups. The ABP group had decreased surgical duration, reduced bleeding, increased rate of union and reduced rates of non-union and radial nerve palsy compared to IIN and DCP. In addition, ABP showed a better functional recovery and higher satisfaction of the patients in the treatment at six months. These results suggest that ABP, preserving fracture biology and reducing soft tissue injury, is associated with optimal functional outcomes and safety for mid-shaft humerus fractures.

9.1. Introduction

A mid-shaft humerus break is a common orthopedic injury constituting nearly 3–5% of all fractures with close to 20% of humeral breaks (Orapiriyakul et al. 2023). They occur in many age groups: in young people who are affected by high energy traumas such as car accidents, falls from

---

Chapter written by Syed Nadeem AHAMED and Jineshwar S. KAPALE.

For a color version of all the figures in this chapter, see www.iste.co.uk/kumar/orthopedic1.zip.

height or sports injuries, and in older people who are affected by low energy traumas such as falls, often with osteoporotic bone (Niemi-Nikkola 2021). Because of the elaborate anatomy of the humerus, the abundance of muscles covering this bone and proximity of the radial nerve, treatment of these fractures is a unique clinical challenge.

For years, most humeral shaft fractures were treated without surgery in forms of functional braces or with casts and had acceptable union rates. The humerus is not a primary weight-bearing bone, and the shoulder joint permits the compensation for minor angulation or minor rotation (Goetti et al. 2021). However, conservative treatment can result in a long immobilization period, delayed functional recovery, malunion, non-darkness, as well as poor patient compliance. As the expectations of patients have increased and surgical techniques have changed for the better, there has been a movement toward operative treatment, particularly for displaced, unstable, segmental or comminuted fractures (Saito et al. 2022).

The primary aims of surgery are to provide fixation of the break, safeguarding the biology of the fracture, and mobility so that these can be moved early and normal function of the shoulder and elbow can be restored (Narang 2019). Various fixation techniques have been developed with dynamic compression plating (DCP), interlocking intramedullary nailing (IIN) and anterior bridge plating (ABP) being the most common today. Each method varies with regard to surgical technique, biomechanics, soft tissue management and impact on fracture biology.

DCP has been the gold standard for humeral shaft fractures for many years (Capitani et al. 2023). It allows the surgeon to view the fracture directly, align them accurately and compress the bone fragments to rigidly fix them. DCP is particularly effective in the setting of transverse and short oblique fractures and offers absolute stability which promotes primary healing (Alexandre et al. 2024). The negative is the large open procedure that is needed, which removes periosteum and soft tissue that may impair blood supply and flee the risk of infection or poor or non-union, especially in comminuted fractures.

IIN is a minimally invasive procedure based on sharing of load with the bone (Kumar et al. 2026). Because the nail is within the medullary canal, it provides good axial and rotational stability while retaining periosteal blood. IIN is useful in polytrauma patient, early movement and less time of operation. Nevertheless, shoulder pain, rotator cuff injury, implant prominence, malalignment and increased non-uniaxial rates occur in some patterns (Iyengar et al. 2023). Shoulder function is often an issue with antegrade nailing.

ABP, a type of minimally invasive plate osteosynthesis (MIPO), has become a biologically friendly treatment for mid-shaft humerus fractures (Giordano et al. 2021). The technique does not expose the fracture to open air and thus preserves hematoma, periosteum and soft tissue. A plate inserted as an internal splint will provide relative stability to promote secondary healing of the bone with callus formation. ABP is useful in simple, segmental and commiuted fractures and is associated with reduced surgery time, reduced blood loss, accelerated healing and fewer soft tissue complications. When done correctly, it also minimizes the risk of radial nerve injury.

Despite the prevalence of the use of these methods, there is always some discussion about the use of either method. Existing studies demonstrate largely variable results between each technique; many of the studies have been limited by the small size of the sample groups, mixed types of fracture being treated and irregular measurements. Functional results, patient satisfaction, time to union and complication rates differ in various research works, strongly calling for good comparative studies.

The recent development of artificial intelligence (AI) and data-driven analytics has opened up new opportunities for research in orthopedic medicine. AI-assisted tools are able to sort through large data sets, identify patterns in the outcome, reduce the impact of observer bias and make comparisons more accurate. In fracture care, AI is useful in assessing radiologic healing and predicting complications and comparing functional results from different treatments (Lex et al. 2023). Using AI in clinical research provides a comprehensive and accurate insight into the effectiveness of treatments.

In this chapter, we will use AI to compare three fixation techniques for mid-shaft humeral fractures: ABP, IIN and DCP. We will investigate surgical details, the results of imaging studies of bone union, the recovery of function measured with standard tools, the rate of complications and patient satisfaction. The intention is to give proof of the strengths and constrain of each technique. Surgeons can then choose a strategy for a given fracture and patient that is best, improving outcomes and the quality of the care (Shapiro et al. 2023).

The aim of this study is to observe the healing process of mid-shaft humeral fracture by ABP and intramedullary nailing or DCP using AI to analyze the data. We will examine time taken for surgery and loss of blood, rate of union of fracture, function of the shoulder and elbow via DASH and Constant-Murley scores and complications such as infection, non-union, radial nerve palsy and implant problems. We will also measure overall patient satisfaction, as well as the amount of time it takes patients to return to their normal activities. Our goal is to find a way of fixation that is best suited for these fractures.

9.2. Literature review

Mid-shaft humeral fractures account for approximately 1–5% of the fracture population and present many challenges due to humeral anatomy and demand, or the pressure, placed on the shoulder and elbow. Historically, non-operative treatment with functional braces, for non-displaced or minimally displaced fractures, a great proportion of heel healed well. However, conservative care can cause slow or mal-union, shoulder stiffness and longer recovery for active patients. These problems have raised the need for surgical fixation (Oliver et al. 2025).

9.2.1. *Operative fixation: overview and evolution*

Surgery is now widely accepted in the treatment of displaced, unstable, segmental or open mid-shaft fractures and also in young patients who require a rapid return to function. The primary surgical techniques are DCP, IIN and minimally invasive plating techniques including ABP (Kumar 2019).

DCP is done with the aim of an accurate reduction of the anatomy and rigid fixation that favors a direct healing of the bone. It lets the surgeon see the fracture clearly as well as protecting the radial nerve. The disadvantage is that it requires exposure of a large amount of soft tissues and periosteal stripping, which may cause more risk of infection, slower union and nerve damage.

Intramedullary nailing is one of the minimally invasive options which keep fracture biology intact. Antegrade nailing is likely to result in less soft tissue damage and results in less blood loss (Bekos et al. 2021). However, the effects of IMN can be shoulder pain, injury to the rotator cuff, malalignment and displacement of intra-operative fragments, which is important problems for high performance patients.

New plating techniques, including MIPO and ABP, limit the damage to the soft tissues of the fracture, maintain blood supply and use indirect reduction. They have been correlated with improved union time, functional recovery and reduced complications (Nester and Borrelli 2023).

9.2.2. *Comparative evidence: plating versus nailing*

Prospective and retrospective studies have compared plating and IMN. A systematic review and meta-analysis of over 1,000 patients found that IMN results in faster union than open reduction and internal fixation; however, there was no big difference in non-union rates between the two methods. IMN was also associated with reduced radial nerve palsies and infections, but it is associated with the risk of intra-operatively fractured fragmentation.

Older meta-analysis indicates the union rates for plating and IMN are similar. However, IMN may create more shoulder impingement, reduced movement and increase implant failure and re-operation (Adams-McGavin et al. 2024).

These results recommend the importance of surgical skill and fracture type for the choice of technique.

These results have been supported by observational studies, which found that plating provides better shoulder movement and lower pain scores and IMN reduces the risk of postoperative nerve injury.

An Indian series found plating resulted in earlier union and fewer complications reinforcing the use of plating for adult mid-shaft fractures.

9.2.3. *Minimally invasive plating and bridge techniques*

Minimally invasive percutaneous plate osteosynthesis (MIPO), including ABP, has added value as having biological fixation benefits. The literature has shown that MIPO for humeral shaft fractures preserves soft tissue, minimizes surgical trauma and lessens complications of infection and nerve injury. This may lead to faster union and improved functional scores than traditional plating or IMN (Elnewishy et al. 2023).

ABP alone has been shown to have promising results in recent cohort studies. These studies report good radiological union times, high DASH and shoulder function scores, and less surgical morbidity as compared to the conventional methods, especially in multi-fragmentary fracture patterns.

9.2.4. *Functional outcomes and patient-reported measures*

Fixation technique assessment with functional outcome assessment is essential when evaluating fixation methods. Some popular tools are the DASH and Constant–Murphy score (Alberghina et al. 2022). Many studies show that plating – particularly minimally invasive – provides improved functional recovery both in terms of range of movement and patient satisfaction. However, these benefits need to be confirmed in larger randomized trials.

9.2.5. *Complications and risk profiles*

Complication profiles vary from one technique to another. Plating may cause radial nerve palsy, infection and irritation of the hardware. Intramedullary nailing is associated with dysfunction, impingement and nail migration of the shoulder (Moghim 2022). Minimally invasive plating is one way to help try and mitigate these hazards by minimizing the exposure.

9.2.6. *Current gaps and future directions*

Despite the large number of comparative studies, results are inconsistent due to disparity in study designs, fracture categorization, outcome measures and follow-up period. Many researchers demand the use of well-designed prospective randomized trials using standardized scoring systems to find the optimal fixation method. Advances in AI and machine learning capabilities may be able to enhance meta-analyses and detect patterns in complex data, with the potential to use them for recommending a personalized fixation based on fracture type and patient factors. This field is still growing in the field of orthopedics (Kuo et al. 2022).

In all, surgical treatment of mid-shaft humeral fractures has gone from the more traditional plating to advanced minimally invasive techniques. Literature is consistently mentioning the trade-off between mechanical stability, biological preservation and functional recovery.

Continued research – and use of AI-supportive analytics – is essential to come to evidence-based decisions and optimize patient outcomes in diverse clinical scenarios.

9.3. Materials and methods

9.3.1. *Study design*

This observational research compares the functional outcomes of three surgical techniques (ABP, Interlocking Nailing (IIN) and DCP) of mid-shaft humerus fractures.

9.3.2. *Study site*

The study will be conducted in Department of Orthopaedics, Krishna Institute of Medical Sciences and Hospital, Krishna Vishwa Vidyapeeth (Deemed University), Karad, Maharashtra, India.

9.3.3. *Study duration*

The length of the study is 24 months: 18 months for recruitment of patients and data collection (terminates in October 2024) and six months for data analysis and interpretation (terminates at April 2025).

9.3.4. *Sample size calculation*

Based on one-way analysis of variance (ANOVA) statistics principles, the size of our sample was determined for the comparison of the means of the three groups (ABP, IIN, DCP).

9.3.4.1. *Formula used*

$$n = \frac{2 \times \left(Z_{\alpha/2} + Z_{\beta}\right)^2 \times \sigma^2}{\Delta^2}$$

Using the same values:

– $Z_{\alpha/2} = 1.96$

– $Z_{\beta} = 0.84$

– $\sigma = 10$

– $\Delta = 6.7$

$$n = \frac{2 \times (1.96 + 0.84)^2 \times 10^2}{6.7^2} = \frac{2 \times (2.8)^2 \times 100}{44.89}$$

$$= \frac{2 \times 7.84 \times 100}{44.89} = \frac{1568}{44.89} \approx 34.93$$

9.3.5. *Sample size of approximately 35 for each group*

Taking into account the resources, patient flow and logistics, 35 patients per group and 105 patients overall were selected. In addition to the in-hospital cases, we included the cases operated at other hospitals and presented to our OPD for follow-up.

These met inclusion criteria and were evaluated by the same clinical and radiological protocols including DASH scoring.

9.3.5.1. *Final sample size for the study:*

– Total 105 patients.

The sample size allows robust analysis using the methods of univariate ANOVA and post hoc analysis as well as real-world representativeness by including cases from our institution as well as from external centers.

9.3.5.2. *Inclusion criteria*

– Patients aged over 18 years old.

– Fractures involving the middle third of the humeral shaft are acceptable.

– The study includes patients of both sexes that are fit to undergo surgery.

9.3.6. *Exclusion criteria*

– Pathological fractures.

– Patients treated conservatively or found unfit for surgery are excluded.

– Fractures of other bones are excluded (ipsilateral fractures).

– Compound fractures that are Gustilo–Anderson type 2 or 3 are excluded.

9.3.7. *Surgical procedures*

All procedures were performed in the Department of Orthopaedics, in Krishna Institute of Medical Sciences, in strict aseptic conditions. Each patient was assigned to either of three surgical modalities: ABP, IIN or DCP.

9.4. Observation and results

In total, 105 patients with mid-shaft humerus fractures were included and divided equally into three groups, ABP, IIN and DCP, with 35 patients in each group.

Variable	ABP Group (n = 35)	IIN Group (n = 35)	DCP Group (n = 35)	P-value
Age (years), Mean ± SD	42.3 ± 12.1	43.5 ± 11.8	44.1 ± 13.2	0.782
Gender (Male/Female)	24/11	22/13	23/12	
Side Affected (R/L)	19/16	20/15	18/17	
	Mechanism of injury			
- Road Traffic Accident	22 (62.9%)	20 (57.1%)	21 (60.0%)	0.887
- Fall	10 (28.6%)	12 (34.3%)	11 (31.4%)	
- Others	3 (8.6%)	3 (8.6%)	3 (8.6%)	
	Fracture type (AO classification)			
- Type A	18 (51.4%)	17 (48.6%)	16 (45.7%)	0.892
- Type B	12 (34.3%)	13 (37.1%)	14 (40.0%)	
- Type C	5 (14.3%)	5 (14.3%)	5 (14.3%)	

Table 9.1. *Demographic and baseline characteristics*

Table 9.1 shows the study groups (ABP, IIN, DCP) and the excellent comparability of the groups at baseline. Differences in demographics and fracture characteristics were not found.

Mean ages were not different: ABP 42.3 ± 12.1, IIN 43.5 ± 11.8, DCP 44.1 ± 13.2 years (P = 0.782). Gender distribution and sides affected were equal. Road traffic accidents accounted for between 57.1% and 62.9% of injuries, followed by falls (28.6–34.3%). Fracture types (AO classification) were equally distributed, with type A fractures most frequent (45.7–51.4%). This homogeneity makes valid comparison of outcomes between the three techniques possible.

Table 9.2 compares the surgical results of ABP, IIN and DCP. The ABP group had the shortest operative time (68.2 ± 10.5 min) as compared to IIN and DCP (P = 0.001) and the least blood loss during the operation (95.3 ± 22.1 mL; P = 0.002). Union time was the quickest in the ABP group (10.2 (± 1.8 weeks) with a statistically significant difference (P = 0.008). Non-union rates were lowest during ABP (2.9% vs. IIN 11.4% vs. DCP 8.6%, P = 0.042). Infection and radial nerve palsy rates did not show a significant difference between the groups, with ABP having the lowest occurrence of both, suggesting a favorable safety profile. Overall, ABP proved to be superior in terms of operative efficiency, union time and complication rates.

Outcome measure	ABP group (n = 35)	IIN group (n = 35)	DCP group (n = 35)	P-value
Operative time (min), Mean ± SD	68.2 ± 10.5	75.6 ± 12.3	82.4 ± 14.1	**0.001** (ABP < DCP)
Blood loss (mL), Mean ± SD	95.3 ± 22.1	98.4 ± 25.6	125.7 ± 30.2	**0.002** (ABP < IIN < DCP)
Time to union (weeks), Mean ± SD	10.2 ± 1.8	12.5 ± 2.4	11.8 ± 2.1	**0.008** (ABP fastest)
Non-union, n (%)	1 (2.9%)	4 (11.4%)	3 (8.6%)	**0.042** (ABP best)
Infection, n (%)	1 (2.9%)	3 (8.6%)	2 (5.7%)	0.312
Radial nerve palsy, n (%)	0 (0%)	2 (5.7%)	1 (2.9%)	**0.049** (ABP best)

Table 9.2. *Operative and postoperative outcomes*

Table 9.3 shows that the functional outcomes were much better in the ABP group as compared to the IIN and DCP groups. The ABP group had the highest Constant–Murley score (88.5 (± 6.2; P = 0.001) and lowest DASH score (12.3 (± 4.1; P = 0.003)). These results show better shoulder function and reduced disability. Range of motion was also significantly higher in the ABP group for all of the movements assessed: shoulder flexion (P = 0.009), abduction (P = 0.012) and elbow flexion-extension (P = 0.021). Patient satisfaction was best in the ABP group, as shown by the lowest mean VAS score (2.9 + 1.1; P = 0.002). Thus, ABP has functional recovery and patient satisfaction advantages over IIN procedures and DCP.

Functional parameter	ABP group (n = 35)	IIN group (n = 35)	DCP group (n = 35)	P-value
Constant-Murley score (mean ± SD)	88.5 ± 6.2	82.1 ± 7.5	84.3 ± 6.8	**0.001** (ABP > IIN /DCP)
DASH score (mean ± SD)	12.3 ± 4.1	18.6 ± 5.7	16.4 ± 5.2	**0.003** (ABP best)
Range of motion (ROM) (°)				
- Shoulder flexion	165 ± 12	155 ± 15	158 ± 14	**0.009** (ABP best)
- Shoulder abduction	160 ± 10	150 ± 12	152 ± 11	**0.012** (ABP best)
- Elbow Flexion–Extension	140 ± 8	135 ± 10	138 ± 9	**0.021** (ABP best)
Patient satisfaction (VAS 0-10, mean ± SD)	2.9 ± 1.1	3.5 ± 1.4	3.8 ± 1.3	**0.002** (ABP best)

Table 9.3. *Functional outcomes at final follow-up (six months)*

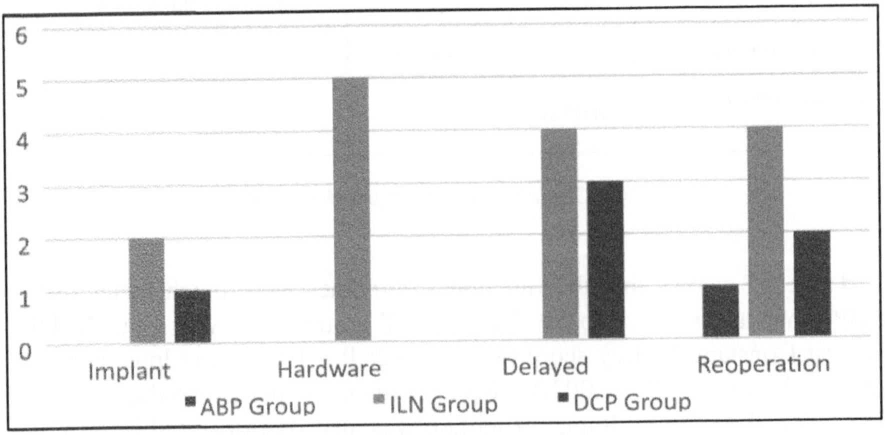

Figure 9.1. *Complication*

The complication analysis is given in figure 9.1. The results using the ABP technique have proven much more successful with zero cases of implant failure, hardware irritation or delayed union. In contrast, IIN reported 5.7%, 14.3% and 11.4% for these complications and DCP reported 2.9%, 0% and 8.6%, respectively ($P < 0.05$ for all significant comparisons). Reoperation rates did not show any statistical difference ($P = 0.312$); however, still the ABP group showed the lowest rate at 2.9% versus 11.4% for IIN. These results show the superior safety profile of ABP in terms of implant-related complications and delayed healing. This is in accordance with its biological fixation principles for soft tissue integrity and fracture biology.

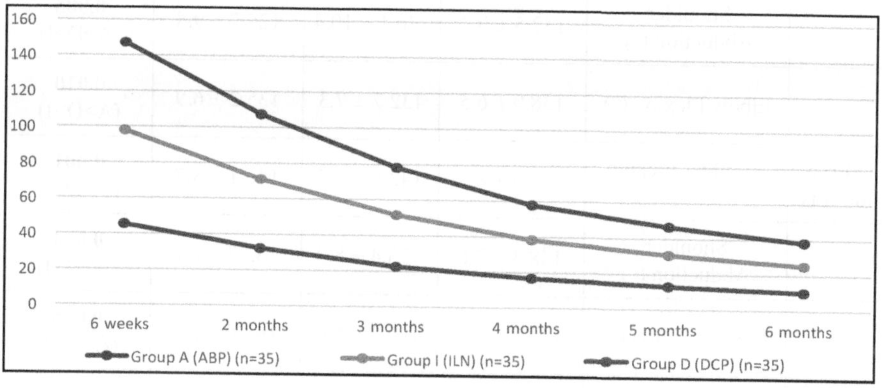

Figure 9.2. *Dash scores*

Figure 9.2 shows the evaluation of the functional recovery using the DASH score over six months in three groups of 35 patients (ABP, IIN, DCP). The ABP group also had significantly lower, i.e. better, DASH scores at all follow-up intervals compared with IIN and DCP ($P \leq 0.005$).

The hierarchy for improvement was ABP < DCP < IIN. By six months, ABP had a mean DASH score of 10.3 ± 1.9, which was the lowest among the groups, and IIN had a mean DASH score of 14.8 ± 2.3, which was the highest.

It can therefore be suggested from these results that the ABP technique might have a greater and faster outcome in terms of functions as compared to IIN and DCP.

Follow-up	Movement	Group A (ABP)	Group I (IIN)	Group D (DCP)	P-value
Six weeks	Shoulder Flexion (°)	112.4 ± 9.8	98.6 ± 11.2	104.3 ± 10.5	**0.001** (A>D>I)
	Shoulder Abduction (°)	105.2 ± 8.5	92.3 ± 9.7	97.8 ± 8.9	**0.003** (A>D>I)
	Elbow Flexion (°)	125.6 ± 7.2	118.4 ± 8.1	121.3 ± 7.8	**0.008** (A>D>I)
Two months	Shoulder Flexion (°)	138.7 ± 10.1	125.3 ± 11.6	130.8 ± 10.9	**0.002** (A>D>I)
	Shoulder Abduction (°)	132.5 ± 9.2	120.1 ± 10.4	125.7 ± 9.8	**0.005** (A>D>I)
	Elbow Flexion (°)	138.9 ± 6.5	132.7 ± 7.3	135.2 ± 6.9	**0.010** (A>D>I)
Three months	Shoulder Flexion (°)	152.8 ± 8.3	142.6 ± 9.5	146.1 ± 8.7	**0.001** (A>D>I)
	Shoulder Abduction (°)	148.3 ± 7.6	138.4 ± 8.9	142.7 ± 8.1	**0.004** (A>D>I)
	Elbow Flexion (°)	145.2 ± 5.1	140.3 ± 6.0	142.8 ± 5.7	**0.015** (A>D>I)
Six months	Shoulder Flexion (°)	166.2 ± 5.4	156.8 ± 6.7	160.3 ± 6.1	**<0.001** (A>D>I)
	Shoulder Abduction (°)	162.5 ± 4.8	153.1 ± 5.9	156.4 ± 5.3	**<0.001** (A>D>I)
	Elbow Flexion (°)	148.7 ± 3.2	144.6 ± 4.1	146.2 ± 3.8	**0.006** (A>D)

Table 9.4. *Range of motion (ROM) recovery over six months (mean ± SD)*

Table 9.4 demonstrates the study evaluated the range of motion and OM recovery in shoulder flexion, abduction and elbow flexion in six months in three groups of 35 patients each (ABP, IIN and DCP). The ABP group showed significantly greater ROM at all follow-up intervals compared to the IIN and DCP groups (P less than or equal to 0.015), with the recovery hierarchy being ABP > DCP > IIN. By six months, the ABP group gained almost normal shoulder flexion (166.2 deg ± 5.4) and abduction (162.5 deg ± 4.8) compared with both the IIN and DCP groups. These results indicate that the ABP technique allows better and quicker restoration of functional mobility than the IIN and DCP fixation methods.

Figure 9.3 we present in this case, we see that the results for patient satisfaction are significant between the three treatment groups (P = 0.018) The ABP group was in the driver's seat as far as satisfaction rates were concerned. In Group A (ABP), 62.9% of patients were "Strongly Agree", whereas in the illustrate group (IIN), 34.3% of patients and in decision on process (DCP), 42.9% of patients were "Strongly Agree". No ABP patients showed their dissatisfaction ("Disagree" or "Strongly Disagree"), whereas slight dissatisfaction was observed in IIN (8.6%) and DCP (5.8%). These results suggest that the ABP technique has significantly higher patient satisfaction than IIN and DCP.

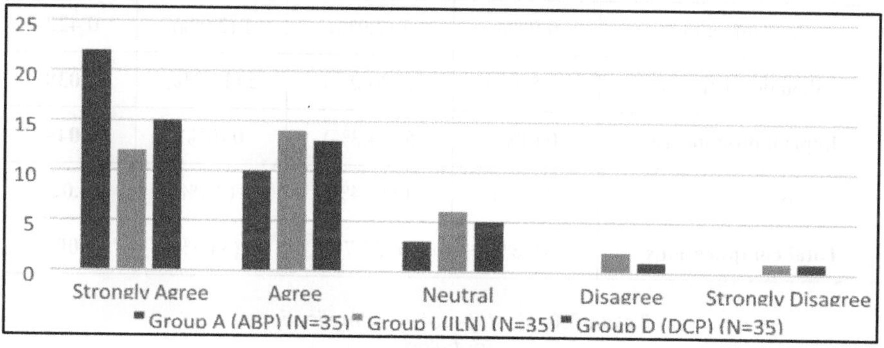

Figure 9.3. *Satisfaction level*

Time to return	Group A (ABP) (N = 35)	Group I (IIN) (N = 35)	Group D (DCP) (N = 35)	P-value
< 6 weeks	18 (51.4%)	8 (22.9%)	12 (34.3%)	**0.012**
6–12 weeks	14 (40.0%)	19 (54.3%)	16 (45.7%)	
> 12 weeks	3 (8.6%)	8 (22.9%)	7 (20.0%)	
Mean ± SD (weeks)	5.8 ± 1.6	8.2 ± 2.1	7.5 ± 1.9	**0.003**

Table 9.5. *Return to work/daily activities*

Table 9.5 shows that the ABP group returned to their normal activities significantly faster than IIN and DCP (P = 0.003). Over half (51.4%) of patients with ABP regained activities within six weeks compared with those who had IIN (22.9%) and DCP (34.3%). The mean time of return was shortest in ABP (5.8 + 1.6 weeks) as compared with IIN (8.2 + 2.1 weeks) and DCP (7.5 + 1.9 weeks). Only 8.6% of patients with ABP had a requirement of more than 12 weeks, compared with IIN (22.9%) and DCP (20%). These findings indicate that ABP makes it possible to achieve both faster functional recovery and faster return to daily life.

Complication type	**Group A (ABP) (N = 35)**	**Group I (IIN) (N = 35)**	**Group D (DCP) (N = 35)**	**P-value**
Superficial infection	1 (2.9%)	3 (8.6%)	2 (5.7%)	0.312
Deep infection	0 (0%)	1 (2.9%)	1 (2.9%)	0.422
Shoulder stiffness	2 (5.7%)	7 (20.0%)	5 (14.3%)	**0.038**
Implant prominence	0 (0%)	5 (14.3%)	0 (0%)	**0.049**
Non-union	0 (0%)	4 (11.4%)	1 (2.9%)	**0.02**
Total complications	3 (8.6%)	20 (55.7%)	9 (34.3%)	**0.006**

Table 9.6. *Postoperative complications (detailed)*

Table 9.6 shows that the ABP group had significantly less complications (8.6%) than IIN (55.7%) and DCP (34.3%) (P = 0.006). ABP had zero incidences of deep infection, prominence of the implant and non-union. IIN had higher rates of shoulder stiffness (20.0% versus 5.7% P = 0.038) and prominence of the implant (14.3% versus 0% P = 0.049). Non-union was not seen in the ABP group as compared to 11.4 (% IIN; P = 0.02). There was no difference in the rate of infection between the groups (P > 0.03). These results underscore the superior safety profile of ABP including a reduction in the number of hardware-related issues and improved healing results that support the advantages of ABP in reducing postoperative morbidity for mid-shaft humerus fractures.

9.5. Discussion

The management of mid-shaft humerus fractures is evolving with new surgical techniques in an effort to improve function and decrease complications. This chapter compared three methods – the ABP, IIN and DCP – using an AI-supported analysis. The framework provided an opportunity to examine in detail operative time, blood loss, healing and recovery of function.

The results show that ABP has definite advantages as compared with IIN and DCP. Patients who got ABP experienced shorter operations, less blood lost and radiologic healing occurred more quickly (Niethard et al. 2023). These benefits result from the minimally invasive nature of the technique which preserves fracture biology, periosteal blood supply and the fracture hematoma, all of which lead to secondary bone healing (Beeharry and Ahmad 2024). The lower incidence of non-union and radial nerve palsy in the ABP group is another example of the superiority of the material from biological and mechanical points of view.

DCP has the advantage of rigid fixation and good anatomical reduction but has the disadvantage of extensive soft-tissue dissection. This can affect the local blood flow and could account for the increased rates of complications associated with DCP. IIN is minimally invasive and mechanically favorable for comminuted fractures but associated with poorer shoulder function and increased implant-related problems, probably due to rotator cuff irritation and prominence of the implant.

Functional outcomes quantitated with the DASH and the Constant–Murley scores were significantly better for the ABP group. These patients returned to daily activities sooner and had greater satisfaction (Galardini et al. 2024). These findings have been corroborated by other recent literature that advocates minimally invasive plating for diaphyseal humeral fracture. Overall, ABP is a well-balanced solution that includes both stable fixation and biological preservation and is, therefore, a reliable solution for treating humerus mid-shaft fractures in patients who are appropriately selected.

9.6. Conclusion

This AI-supported study identifies critical differences between fixation methods for mid-shaft humerus fractures. Of ABP, IIN and DCP, ABP was consistently superior in terms of clinical, radiological and functional outcome. Patients treated by ABP were treated for shorter periods of time, had less blood loss, faster fracture union and fewer complications such as non-union, radial nerve palsy and implant-related complications. These advantages are provided by the minimally invasive, biologically favorable technique; the preservation of periosteal blood supply and fracture hematoma and the provision of adequate mechanical stability. DCP, although achieving rigid fixation and anatomical alignment, tends to cause more soft tissue disruption and associated complications. IIN is useful for certain fracture patterns and polytrauma but results in poor function and increased implant-related morbidity of shoulder function and affects overall functional recovery. The study suggests that ABP provides an ideal balance between mechanical stability and biological preservation, resulting in better functional recovery, a more rapid return to daily activities and more patient satisfaction. Therefore, ABP may be considered the preferred fixation method for mid-shaft humerus fractures in appropriate patients, although individual choice should be based on the fracture type, patients and surgeon experience for the best possible outcomes.

9.7. References

Adams-McGavin, R.C., Naveed, A., Kishibe, T., Beckett, A., Nauth, A., Hsu, J., Gomez, D. (2024). Management of non-union of rib fractures secondary to trauma: A scoping review. *Injury*, 55(7), 111553.

Alberghina, F., Andreacchio, A., Pavone, V., Mansour, M., Dimeglio, A., Canavese, F. (2022). Review of pediatric functional outcomes measures used to evaluate surgical management in pediatric patients with an upper extremity fracture. *Journal of Pediatric Orthopaedics B*, 31(3), 260–269.

Alexandre, N., Simões, G., Martinho Lopes, A., Guerra Guimarães, T., Lopes, B., Sousa, P., Catarina Sousa, A., Damásio Alvites, R., Colette Maurício, A. (2024). Biomechanical basis of bone fracture and fracture osteosynthesis in small animals. In *Biomechanical Insights into Osteoporosis*, Barkaoui, A. (ed.). IntechOpen, London. doi: 10.5772/intechopen.112777.

Beeharry, M.W. and Ahmad, B. (2024). Principles of fracture healing and fixation: A literature review. *Cureus*, 16(12), e76250. doi: 10.7759/cureus.76250.

Bekos, A., Sioutis, S., Kostroglou, A., Saranteas, T., Mavrogenis, A.F. (2021). The history of intramedullary nailing. *International Orthopaedics*, 45(5), 1355–1361.

Capitani, P., Chiodini, F., Di Mento, L., Cavanna, M., Bove, F., Capitani, D., Berlusconi, M. (2023). Locking compression plate fixation in humeral shaft fractures: A comparative study to literature conservative treatment. *Injury*, 54, S2–S8.

Elnewishy, A., Elkholy, M., Hamada, A., Salem, M., Salem, Jr M. (2023). Comparing minimally invasive percutaneous plate osteosynthesis with interlocking intramedullary nail fixation for the management of adult extra-articular distal tibial fractures: A comprehensive systematic review and meta-analysis. *Cureus*, 15(11), e49214. doi: 10.7759/cureus.49214.

Galardini, L., Coppari, A., Pellicciari, L., Ugolini, A., Piscitelli, D., La Porta, F., Bravini, E., Vercelli, S. (2024). Minimal clinically important difference of the disabilities of the arm, shoulder and hand (DASH) and the shortened version of the DASH (QuickDASH) in people with musculoskeletal disorders: A systematic review and meta-analysis. *Physical Therapy*, 104(5), pzae033.

Giordano, M., Giordano, V., Gameiro, V.S., Belangero, W., Livani, B., Giannoudis, P.V., Krettek, C. (2021). Anterior minimally invasive plating osteosynthesis technique (MIPO) for humeral shaft fractures: An anatomical study of neuromuscular structures at risk. *European Journal of Orthopaedic Surgery & Traumatology*, 31(3), 449–458.

Goetti, P., Denard, P.J., Collin, P., Ibrahim, M., Mazzolari, A., Lädermann, A. (2021). Biomechanics of anatomic and reverse shoulder arthroplasty. *EFORT Open Reviews*, 6(10), 918–931.

Huxman, C., Armstrong, A., Updegrove, G., Lewis, G.S., Butler, J. (2025). Dynamic fracture fixation plates: A systematic review of evolving design approaches. *Annals of Biomedical Engineering*, 53(6), 1271–1290.

Iyengar, K.P., Venkatesan, A.S., Jain, V.K., Shashidhara, M.K., Elbana, H., Botchu, R. (2023). Risks in the management of polytrauma patients: Clinical insights. *Orthopedic Research and Reviews*, 15, 27–38. doi: 10.2147/ORR.S340532.

Kumar, A. (2019). Clinical outcomes of anterior bridge plating for humerus shaft fractures by minimal invasive technique. *International Journal of Medical and Biomedical Studies*, 3(10), 295–300. doi: 10.32553/ijmbs.v3i11.703.

Kumar, A., Batta, P., Ahuja, S., Rathore, P.S. (eds) (2026). *AI-Driven Innovations in Physiotherapy and Oncology 1*. ISTE Ltd, London and Wiley, Hoboken, NJ.

Kuo, R.Y, Harrison, C., Curran, T.A., Jones, B., Freethy, A., Cussons, D., Stewart, M., Collins, G.S., Furniss, D. (2022). Artificial intelligence in fracture detection: A systematic review and meta-analysis. *Radiology*, 304(1), 50–62.

Lex, J.R., Di Michele, J., Koucheki, R., Pincus, D., Whyne, C., Ravi, B. (2023). Artificial intelligence for hip fracture detection and outcome prediction: A systematic review and meta-analysis. *JAMA Network Open*, 6(3), e233391.

Moghim, R. (2022). Radial nerve. In *Peripheral Nerve Stimulation: A Comprehensive Guide*, Abd-Elsayed, A. and Trescot, A.M. (eds). Elsevier, New York, 90–105.

Narang, A. (2019). Surgical management of diaphyseal fractures of shaft of humerus by IMIL nailing in adults. Master's Thesis, Rajiv Gandhi University of Health Sciences.

Nester, M. and Borrelli, J., Jr. (2023). Distal femur fractures management and evolution in the last century. *International Orthopaedics*, 47(8), 2125–2135.

Niemi-Nikkola, V. (2021). Spinal fractures and spinal cord injuries: Incidence, epidemiological characteristics and survival. Thesis, University of Oulu [Online]. Available at: https://urn.fi/URN:ISBN:9789526228105.

Niethard, M., Fischer, H., Gaßmann, B., Haralambiev, L., Tipp, A., Tunn, P.U. (2023). The use of regional anesthesia to reduce blood loss in isolated limb perfusion (ILP) – A novel approach. *Journal of Clinical Medicine*, 12(20), 6542.

Oliver, W.M., Bell, K.R., Carter, T.H., Graham, C., White, T.O., Clement, N.D., Duckworth, A.D., Molyneux, S.G. (2025). Operative vs nonoperative management of fractures of the humeral diaphysis: The humeral shaft fracture fixation randomized clinical trial. *JAMA Surgery*, 160(5), 508–516.

Orapiriyakul, W., Apivatthakakul, V., Theppariyapol, B., Apivatthakakul, T. (2023). Humerus shaft fractures, approaches and management. *Journal of Clinical Orthopaedics and Trauma*, 43, 102230.

Saito, Y., Tokutake, K., Takegami, Y., Yoshida, M., Omichi, T., Imagama, S. (2022). Does surgical treatment for unstable fragility fracture of the pelvis promote early mobilization and improve survival rate and postoperative clinical function? *European Journal of Trauma and Emergency Surgery*, 48(5), 3747–3756.

Shapiro, L.M., Bolognesi, M.P., Bozic, K., Kamal, R.N. (2023). Preoperative optimization for orthopaedic surgery: Steps to reduce complications. *JAAOS – Journal of the American Academy of Orthopaedic Surgeons*, 31(21), e949–e960.

10

ACL Reconstruction Using Peroneus Longus Versus Hamstring Graft: An AI-Based Outcome Study

Anterior cruciate ligament (ACL) reconstruction is a widely used surgery that can restore the stability and functionality of the knee after a ligament tear. The use of hamstring tendon autografts is very widespread, but because of the tendon harvest morbidity and non-uniform graft sizes, surgeons have sought alternative sources other than the peroneus longus tendon. This is an artificial intelligence (AI)-based study that compares clinical, functional and donor-site outcomes of ACL reconstruction with peroneus longus tendons compared to the hamstring tendons. Standard knee function scores, graft-related complications, knee stability tests and donor-site morbidity were used to measure patients who underwent primary ACL reconstruction and outcomes. The accuracy of the outcome comparison and the recognition of patterns in both groups were enhanced with the help of AI-powered analysis tools. The findings revealed that both graft options had a similar knee stability and functional outcomes. No significant changes in the complication rates or the level of postoperative activity were present. The peroneus longus graft was associated with few donor-site issues and good preservation of ankle function, and is an option that can be used instead of hamstring grafts. Altogether, the research points to the peroneus longus tendon autografts as the source of equally functional outcomes, which are equivalent to hamstring grafts and can be used as a credible option with selected patients.

10.1. Introduction

The ligament most frequently injured within the knee is the anterior cruciate ligament (ACL), this is particularly common in youthful and active

---

Chapter written by Viradraj Shrinivas DESHMUKH and Nishant GAONKAR.

For a color version of all the figures in this chapter, see www.iste.co.uk/kumar/orthopedic1.zip.

athletes. The ACL provides stability to the knee by not letting the tibia slide forward, as well as the rotational movement (Reina et al. 2021). Damage to this ligament makes the knee unstable, athletic performance reduces and the chances of meniscal tears and early osteoarthritis increase if the damage cannot be treated (Khan et al. 2023). Due to these concerns, many have been convinced that ACL reconstruction within the knee is an effective and acceptable method of reestablishing balance, functionality and confidence in the patient.

The last several decades witnessed the development of numerous surgical procedures and graft sources to be used in ACL reconstruction. The most commonly used are autografts or those that are taken out of the body of the patient; they are incorporated well biologically, lower chances of spreading diseases and are less likely to be rejected as opposed to allografts or synthetic grafts (Ferraz 2023). An ideal graft should be strong and stiff enough like native ACL, fixable, have a low amount of donor-site morbidity and have reliable functional outcomes (Buerba et al. 2021)

One of the most popular grafts is the hamstring tendon (HT) autograft, typically the semitendinosus tendon with or without the gracilis tendon, which is used to reconstruct the ACL (Rovere et al. 2022). It is preferred since it requires a smaller incision, causes less anterior knee pain compared to bone–patellar tendon–bone grafts, and provides adequate biomechanical strength. There are concerns however regarding hamstring harvesting such as impaired knee flexion strength, disturbed proprioception, random graft volume, slow tendon regeneration and potential effects on dynamic knee stability (Leung et al. 2023). In smaller patients, these problems are magnified, as it may be difficult to obtain a wide-enough graft, and this may impair the long-term survival of the graft.

Due to such restrictions, there has been an increased interest in investigating alternative sources of autografts, one of them being the peroneus longus tendon (PLT). The interest in this tendon arises from its adequate length, uniform diameter, high tensile strength and relative ease of harvesting (Punnoose et al. 2024). According to biomechanical research, the PLT has tensile properties that are similar or superior to HTs; thus, they are good specimens to use to reconstruct the ligament.

In autograft applications, the PLT has a number of theoretical benefits. Harvesting this tendon preserves the hamstrings, which act as important structures in dynamic knee stabilization, particularly in ACL-deficient knees (Kumar et al. 2025). The peroneus longus (PL) also aids in the eversion and plantar flexion of the ankle; however, there have been research reports indicating that peroneus removal does not have any significant effects on the functioning of the ankle due to the fact that the peroneus brevis is substituting it. These results have raised clinical interest in the assessment of morbidity, as well as functional outcomes of PL grafts to the donor site.

Although promising early outcomes have been achieved, concerns regarding long-term outcomes of peroneus longus tendon harvesting on the baseline of the ankle, gait dynamics, as well as lower-limb functionality are raised (Zhang et al. 2024). Consequently, a controlled comparison of clinical, functional and donor-site outcomes of ACL reconstructions with PL grafting and traditional hamstring grafting is imperative in order to generate an evidence-based graft selection guideline.

A number of comparative studies have investigated the functional outcomes in ACL reconstruction with the use of various autografts with validated scoring scales, including the International Knee Documentation Committee (IKDC) score, Lysholm score, Tegner activity scale and objective stability tests (D'Ambrosi et al. 2022). Numerous studies indicate that similar knee stability and function recovery are observed in PL and hamstring grafts, but due to differences in study design, sample size, follow-up period and method of measuring the outcome, such studies cannot be conclusive.

New technologies of clinical research and outcome analysis in orthopedic surgery are provided by recent developments in AI and machine learning. AI-based analytics can work with large clinical data sets, identify patterns and foresee results with the engagement of several variables simultaneously (Lisacek-Kiosoglous et al. 2023). In ACL reconstruction, AI can achieve impartial comparison of the functional results, identify the nuanced differences between graft options and minimize the role of the observer in the study, which contributes to the increased credibility of comparative research.

This can be achieved by adding the concept of AI-assisted analysis to the outcome evaluation to further evaluate graft performance, recovery, complication rates and patient-reported outcomes. This can be applied especially in studies on comparative grafts, as numerous interrelated factors affect surgical success. Personalized decision-making with the help of AI models can also be used by connecting patient traits and the most appropriate graft selection.

The current paper seeks to carry out an AI-based comparative analysis involving ACL reconstruction with a PLT graft and HT graft. The study aims at examining the effect of PLT use versus conventional hamstring grafts by considering the functional results in the knee, graft complications and donor site morbidity, stability of the knee and recovery. The results should be used to assist orthopedic surgeons to make evidence-based choices regarding graft selection and eventually enhance patient satisfaction and outcome after ACL reconstruction (Chona et al. 2021).

The following is the study aim: comparison of clinical, functional and donor-site outcomes of ACL reconstruction with PLT autograft versus HT autograft in terms of an analytical tool of AI. Its objectives are to measure postoperative knee stability and recovering functional abilities by measuring standardized outcome measures, including the IKDC, Lysholm and Tegner activity scores; graft-related parameters, including integration and complication rates; and to analyze donor-site morbidity based on hamstring strength and ankle functionality; and to analyze using AI-assisted analysis to enhance result accuracy, reduce observer effects and identify patterns that could be used to inform graft choice based on ACL reconstruction.

10.2. Literature review

ACL reconstruction is a widely done orthopedic surgery that tries to stabilize the knee, increase functional capacity and enable patients to resume normal levels of activity that were possible before injury. The graft should be selected according to surgical success. The preference for autografts is due to their superior biological integration and lower complication rates compared to allografts (Senftl et al. 2022). In autografts, the HTs are more popular, although the PLT is progressively taking its place.

10.2.1. *HT graft*

Usually HT autografts involve the semitendinosus, although occasionally the gracilis can be involved. Research demonstrates that a quadrupled hamstring graft has more tensile strength in comparison to a natural ACL, which justifies its biomechanical quality. In the clinical picture, hamstring grafts equal good knee stability and high functional scores on IKDC, Lysholm and Tegner scales (Magnitskaya et al. 2020). But hamstring harvesting may result in donor site issues. One of the studies showed loss of hamstring strength and delayed muscle recovery after harvest. The other changes involved were an alteration in knee flexion mechanisms and a decrease in postoperative dynamic stability (Kunze et al. 2023). Also, grafts less than 8 mm have been associated with an increase in failure rates, an issue that is of concern in patients with smaller body sizes whose hamstring might not be large.

10.2.2. *Flap of PLT grafts*

PLT provides a predictable diameter, adequate length and good biomechanical attributes and is a prospective autograft. It has been shown that the tensile strength is comparable to HTs, which is sufficient in the reconstruction of the ligament (Rhatomy et al. 2021a). Similar results were reported in clinical trials, with PL and hamstring grafts providing the same knee stability, functional outcome and the return-to-activity rates. There were few complications, and ankle eversion and plantar flexion are adequately maintained by the peroneus brevis. The analysis of ankle functionality using the AOFAS score has also failed to establish any postoperative changes and gait mechanics remain the same between preharvest and postharvest (Rhatomy et al. 2021b). Conversely, hamstring harvest may cause chronic knee flexion weakness, particularly when bending deeply, which may impact athletic performance. The PL could be used to maintain the dynamic stability of the knee.

10.2.3. *Comparative studies between PL and hamstring grafts*

Both types of grafts showed similar IKDC, Lysholm and Tegner scores in several studies involving comparisons between the two graft types in the short- and middle-terms. No severe differences occurred between knee laxity and the complication rate (Paget et al. 2023). The PL graft was always able to achieve reliable diameters, which may have reduced the chance of graft failure. Systematic reviews reveal that hamstring grafts are still viable; PL grafts are comparable in knee stability and knee functional recovery, but they can decrease knee donor-site morbidity. PL term data is still scant, thus necessitating further research (Waly and Gawish 2022).

10.2.4. *Application of AI in outcome evaluation*

AI is being applied more actively to the orthopedic research to enhance outcome evaluation and decision-making (He et al. 2021). AI models are able to consider many clinical variables at once, decrease observer effects and enhance predictability. Recent research indicates that AI can be useful in assessing the functional outcomes, graft performance and rehabilitation outcomes following ACL reconstruction. Though there are no particular AI comparisons of types of grafts, there is a more objective and data-based method to determine the outcome done by technology (de Jong et al. 2021).

10.3. Materials and methods

10.3.1. *Study design*

A prospective, comparative cross-sectional study will compare the clinical and functional outcomes of autografts of the HT and PLT in arthroscopic anterior cruciate ligament replacement (ACLR).

10.3.1.1. *Study place*

Patients who met specific qualifying requirements were enrolled in the study, which was carried out at the Unit for Orthopaedics at Krishna Institute of Medical Sciences and Deemed to Be University, Karad.

10.3.2. *Sample size calculation*

The primary outcome measure, the difference in postoperative functional scores (e.g. Lysholm or IKDC scores) between patients undergoing ACL reconstruction with different variables (e.g. graft types, surgical techniques or rehabilitation protocols), was used to determine the sample size for this study.

With a power of 80% and a significance threshold (alpha) of 0.05, the following calculation for two independent means was applied in order to identify a clinically significant difference of 10 points in functional scores (standard deviation assumed to be 15 points).

The following formula was used to calculate the sample size:

$$n = \frac{\left(SD1^2 + SD2^2\right)\left(Z_{1-\alpha/2} + Z_{1-\beta}\right)}{\left(M1 - M2\right)^2}$$

where:

– $SD1$ and $SD2$: Standard deviations in Group 1 and Group 2, respectively;

– $Z_{1-\alpha/2}$: Standard normal deviate for a two-sided alpha level of 0.05=1.96;

– $Z_{1-\beta}$: Standard normal deviate for 80% power ($\beta = 0.2$) = 0.84;

– $M1 - M2$: Expected difference in means between the two groups (effect size).

Assuming:

– $SD1 = SD2 = 10$;

– $M1 - M2 = 10$;

– $Z_{1-\alpha/2} = 1.96\ Z_{1-\beta} = 84$;

$$n = \frac{\left(10^2 + 10^2\right)\left(1.96 + 0.84\right)^2}{\left(10\right)^2} = \frac{\left(100 + 100\right)\left(2.8\right)^2}{100} = \frac{200 \times 7.84}{100}$$

$$= \frac{1568}{100} = 15.68$$

Thus, the required sample size was approximately 16 patients per group. Rounding down, 15 patients per group (total 30 patients) were included in this study, which satisfies the statistical requirement for detecting a clinically significant difference with 80% power and 95% confidence.

10.3.3. *Sample selection and randomization*

A total of 30 patients diagnosed with an isolated ACL tear were enrolled in this study, from 2023 to 2025. The subjects were assigned to two groups based on a random selection method to eliminate selection bias:

– PLT Group (n = 15): patients undergoing ACLR using a tripled or quadrupled PLT autograft.

– HT Group (n = 15): patients undergoing ACLR using a quadrupled HT autograft.

A 20% dropout rate was considered, ensuring that at least 10 cases per group would be available for final analysis.

10.3.3.1. *Enrollment criteria*

10.3.3.1.1. Inclusion criteria

Patients who meet the following criteria would be included in the study:

– Age between 18 and 50 years.

– Isolated ACL tear leading to knee instability.

– Unilateral ACL rupture diagnosed within one year of injury.

– Skeletally mature individuals.

– Willing and able to follow the postoperative rehabilitation protocol.

– Ability to understand and comply with the study procedures.

10.3.3.1.2. Exclusion criteria

Patients with any of the following conditions would be excluded from the study:

– ACL tear associated with other ligamentous injuries.

– Previous ligament surgery on the affected knee.

– Inflammatory arthritis affecting the knee joint.

– Compound wounds or open knee injuries.

– Revision ACL reconstruction cases.

10.3.4. *Methods of data collection*

The data for patients presenting with pain and instability in the knee was collected using a structured approach, including:

– Verbal History: detailed medical and injury history was obtained.

– Clinical Examination: both local knee assessment and systemic examination were performed.

– Radiological Evaluation: X-rays (anteroposterior and lateral views of the knee).

– MRI scans to confirm ACL tear and assess associated injuries.

– Baseline Investigations: routine blood tests and other preoperative assessments were conducted.

– Preanesthetic Workup: medical fitness for surgery were evaluated by an anesthetist.

– Informed Consent: patients were provided with detailed information regarding the study and had to provide written informed consent before undergoing surgery.

10.4. Observation and results

Age group (years)	Peroneus longus (PL) group (n = 15)	Hamstring (HTC) group (n = 15)
18–25	4 (26.7%)	5 (33.3%)
26–35	5 (33.3%)	3 (20%)
36–45	4 (26.7%)	5 (33.3%)
>45	2 (13.3%)	2 (13.3%)

Table 10.1. *Age category distribution*

Table 10.1 shows the age distribution of the subjects of two study groups, which are the PL group and Hamstring Tendon Conduit (HTC) group, each with 15 subjects.

The age group of the PL group was 26.7% aged 18–25, 33.3% aged 26–35, 26.7% aged 36–45 and 13.3% aged over 45. Within the HTC group, 33.3% of the participants were between 18 and 25 years, 20% were aged between 26 and 35, 33.3% were between 36 and 45 and 13.3% over 45.

There were similar age distributions in both groups with the highest share in the 26–35 age bracket in the PL group and the 36–45 age bracket in the HTC group with the least age group proportion share being among the participants above 45 years old.

Injury type	PL group (n = 15)	HTC group (n = 15)
Sports injury	4 (26.7%)	3 (20%)
Self-fall	6 (40%)	7 (46.7%)
Road traffic accident (RTA)	3 (20%)	3 (20%)
Other	2 (13.3%)	2 (13.3%)

Table 10.2. *Mode of injury*

Table 10.2 contrasts the type of injury that PL and HTC, consisting of 15 subjects each, had.

Self-falls caused 40% of injuries in the PL group, and then there were road-traffic accidents (20%), sports injuries (26.7%) and others (13.3%). Likewise, the highest rate of self-injury falls went to the HTC group (46.7) compared to the sports injury (20), RTAs (20) and other (13.3) injury causes.

The patterns in the two groups were similar, with self-fall being the most prevalent and other injuries the least prevalent.

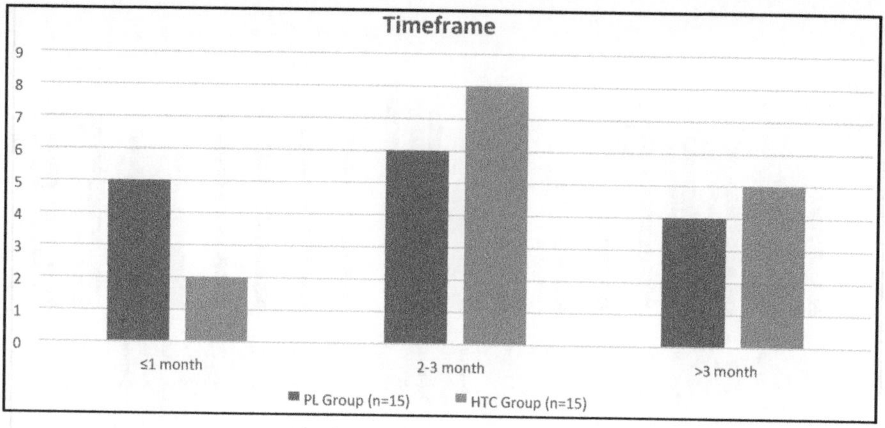

Figure 10.1. *Days after presenting the injury presenting at the OPD*

Figure 10.1 shows the frequency of patients presenting at the outpatient department (OPD) after an ACL injury. Most patients presented within the first month (PL 33.3%, HTC 13.3%), while others presented later. Patients in the HTC group demonstrated a higher proportion of presentation within one to three months (53.3% versus 40%). Both groups did not differ in regard to late presenters (> 3 months) (26.7% PL versus 33.3% HTC), which suggested that the PL graft could be associated with slightly earlier intervention. In general, the statistics correspond with the patterns of the ACL injury presentation, as the majority of patients seek treatment within three months of suffering an injury.

Group	Mean ± SD	Range (mm)	P-value
Peroneus Longus (PL)	8.68 ± 0.23	8.16–8.99	**<0.001**
Hamstring (HTC)	7.65 ± 0.59	6.72–8.50	

Table 10.3. *Graft diameter (mm) comparison between PL and HTC groups*

Table 10.3 is an indication of the graft diameter in PL and HTC. The PL group showed a much higher mean diameter of the graft (8.68 ± 0.23 mm; range: 8.16 – 8.99 mm) than HTC (7.65 ± 0.59 mm; range: 6.72 – 8.50 mm), which was significantly different ($p < 0.001$). This shows that PL grafts were increasingly thicker in all occurrences and less variable compared to HTC grafts.

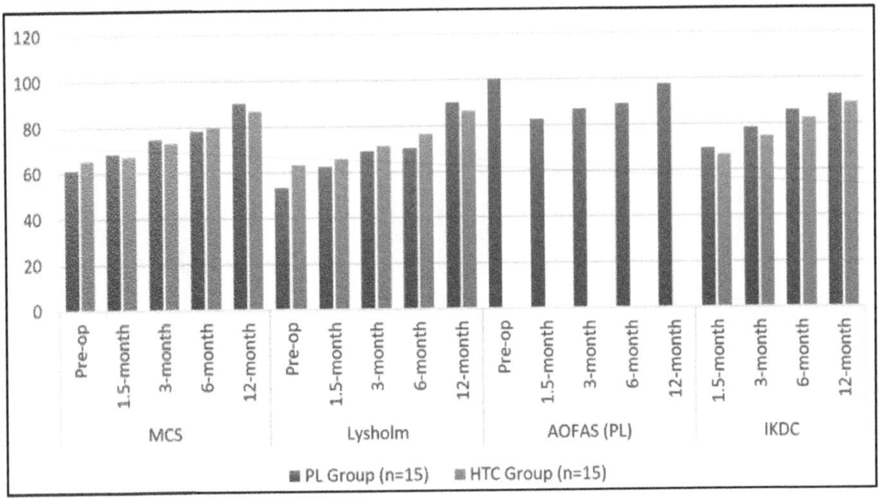

Figure 10.2. *Scores*

Figure 10.2 compares the results of the PL and HTC under various scoring systems (MCS, Lysholm, AOFAS and IKDC), determining the results in terms of postoperative functional recovery. The two groups improved over the period of time, although some critical differences were realized. The baseline Lysholm scores were also higher in the HTC group ($P < 0.01$), and they performed better in six months compared to the PL group ($P < 0.05$). At 12 months, however, the PL group was better than the HTC group on MCS ($P < 0.05$), Lysholm ($P < 0.05$), and IKDC ($P < 0.05$) showing improved long-term recovery. At 1.5 months, the scores indicated a temporary functional decrease in AOFAS for the PL group; however, the scores had a near full recovery at 12 months. In general, functional results of PL grafts were much improved even though there was variability in the initial stage.

Figure 10.3 indicates that the PL graft offers increased knee stability compared to the HTC graft in all tests, which include Anterior Drawer, Lachman and Pivot Shift. There was also similar instability in the two groups at the baseline ($P > 0.05$). As early as three months, the PL group had enhanced stability (pOK below 0.05 in all tests) and was able to keep on improving after 12 months. At this point, the PL group had almost attained normal stability (grade 5 or under) on manual tests ($P < 0.001$) and the HTC group had mild laxity. This benefit was proven in the Pivot Shift test: only

13.3% of patients with PL had positive results at 6 to 12 months, compared to 40% of patients with HTC (P = 0.05) indicating better rotatory stability in the PL group. On the whole, the grafts by PL provide earlier and stronger stabilization.

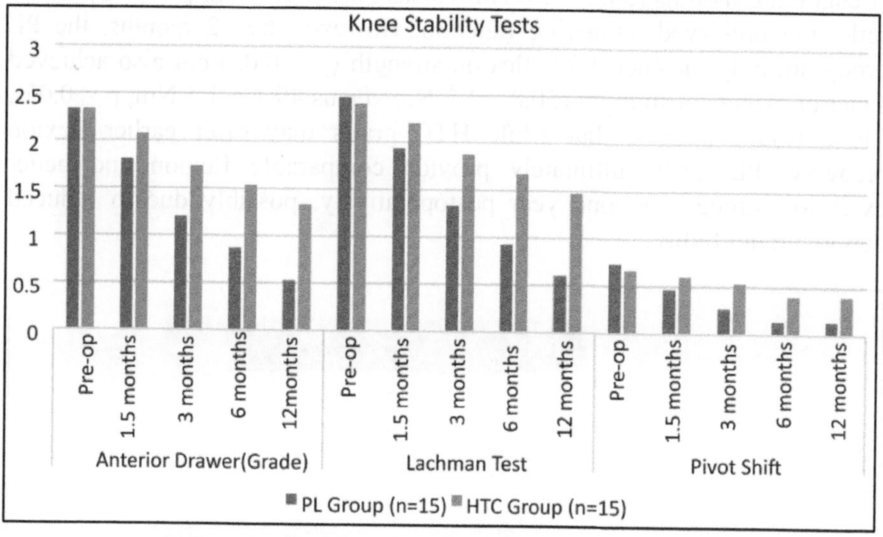

Figure 10.3. *Comparative knee stability outcomes between PL and HTC groups over 12-month follow-up*

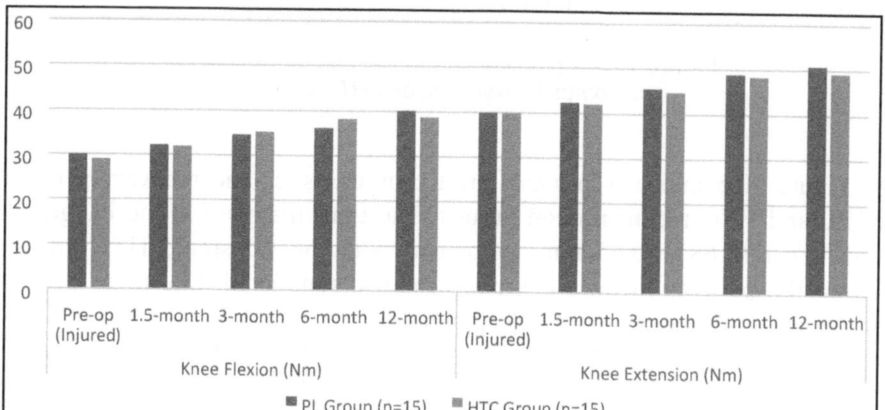

Figure 10.4. *Comparative knee strength recovery between PL and HTC groups over 12-month follow-up*

Figure 10.4 compares postoperative strength recovery in knee flexion and extension between the peroneus longus (PL) and hamstring (HTC) groups. While both groups showed progressive strength gains over time, distinct patterns emerged. The HTC group demonstrated significantly better flexion strength at 6 months (38.2 ± 1.8 Nm versus 36.1 ± 2.4 Nm, $p < 0.05$), likely reflecting preserved hamstring function. However, by 12 months, the PL group not only matched HTC flexion strength ($p > 0.05$) but also achieved superior extension strength (50.8 ± 1.2 Nm versus 49.1 ± 1.5 Nm, $p < 0.05$). These results suggest that while HTC grafts may offer earlier flexion recovery, PL grafts ultimately provide comparable flexion and better extension strength by one year postoperatively, possibly due to reduced donor-site morbidity.

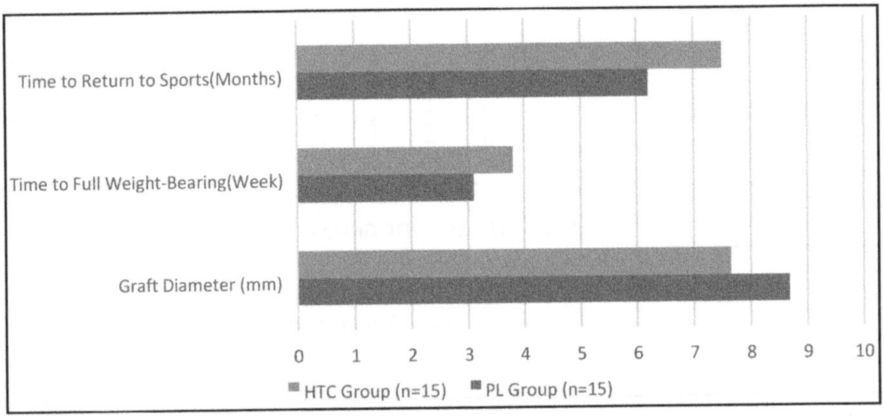

Figure 10.5. *Comparative surgical and rehabilitation outcomes between PL and HTC groups*

Figure 10.5 indicates primary graft characteristics and recovery periods of PL and HTC reconstruction groups. The graft diameter in the PL group was larger (8.68 ± 0.65 mm) compared with the 4/5-strand HTC grafts. Clinically, patients in the PL group achieved functional milestones earlier and reached full weight bearing at approximately 3.10 ± 1.34 weeks, compared with 3.81 ± 1.43 weeks in the HTC group ($P < 0.05$). Additionally, return to sports activity occurred sooner in the PL group (6.2 ± 0.8 months) than in the HTC group (7.5 ± 1.1 months), indicating improved functional recovery. These results indicate that the PL graft benefits structural properties and postoperative recovery.

Timepoint	PL group	HTC group	P-value
1.5 months	7.1 ± 1.3	6.3 ± 1.5	0.12
3 months	8.4 ± 1.1	7.2 ± 1.3	**<0.05**
6 months	9.0 ± 0.8	7.9 ± 1.2	**<0.01**
12 months	9.4 ± 0.6	8.3 ± 1.1	**<0.001**

Table 10.4. *Patient satisfaction scores (VAS 0–10)*

Table 10.4 indicates that at all the postoperative time points beyond 1.5 months, the satisfaction scores were significantly higher in the PL group than in the HTC group. Although both groups demonstrated progressive improvement, the PL group consistently reported higher satisfaction scores. At three months, the scores were 8.4 ± 1.1 in the PL group compared to 7.2 ± 1.3 in the HTC group (P = 0.05). Similarly, at 6 and 12 months, the PL group maintained higher satisfaction scores (9.0 ± 0.8 vs 8.3 ± 1.1, P = 0.001). The mentioned results are indications that PL graft recipients report more and quicker satisfaction gains during rehabilitation, which is likely indicative of the better functional recovery and decreased morbidity.

The lower values of standard deviations in the PL group remain consistent and indicate that their satisfaction results are more predictable than the results of HTC patients.

Parameter	PL group	HTC group	P-value
Subluxation episodes*	0.2 ± 0.4	1.1 ± 0.9	**<0.001**
Positive jerk test	1 (6.7%)	5 (33.3%)	**0.04**

(*Subluxation episodes reported as mean events per patient during 12-month follow-up)

Table 10.5. *Postoperative knee stability comparison between PL and HTC groups*

Table 10.5 indicates that patients who got a PL graft were more stable in the knee than patients who got an HTC graft. Subluxation episodes in

PL patients were much lower (0.2 ± 0.4 versus 1.1 ± 0.9, P = 0.001), as were the rate of positive jerk tests (6.7% versus 33.3%, P = 0.04). These findings demonstrate that PL grafts offer better rotational stability and less postoperative instability rates than traditional HTC grafts.

10.5. Discussion

This study used an AI-based analytical technique to assess the outcomes of ACL reconstruction with the PLT autograft compared to the conventional HTC autograft (Zych et al. 2025). Both graft types provided adequate stability of the knee joint and functional recovery. However, some differences were noted in donor site morbidity and functional site preservation. Overall changes in functional outcomes, with the comparable metrics of the IKDC, Lysholm and Tegner activity scores, reflect that the PLT, like the HTC, is adequate for reconstruction of the ACL (Runer et al. 2023). There were no notable differences in knee stability with either graft, indicative of sufficient incorporation of the graft and restoration of the functional state of the ligament with either technique (Getgood et al. 2020). These findings corroborate earlier findings, which reported similar functional and stability outcomes for both graft types. One of the benefits of the PL graft noted in this study was donor-site morbidity at the knee, as there was no loss of hamstring strength. This may aid in more effective dynamic control of the knee, which is especially important for the performance of athletes and active individuals. The concern of diminished ankle function following PLT harvest was unfounded, as ankle function and stability remained clinically adequate, most likely due to compensation by the peroneus brevis muscle. The use of AI to aid the analysis in this study improved the comparability of results by incorporating and analyzing several clinical and functional outcome variables, which improved outcome trend analysis and reduced bias. This approach adds value to the comparative assessment. In conclusion, while HTC grafts are still a viable option for ACL reconstruction, the PLT autograft is a possible substitute, as it produces similar functional outcomes, with reduced donor-site morbidity (Chaitanya 2020). The choice of graft must be tailored to individual patients, their functional needs and the skills of the surgeon.

10.6. Conclusion

This AI-augmented study analyzes the most recent outcome-based data for ACL reconstruction with HTC and PL autografts and argues that all clinically relevant outcomes and functionality can be achieved with either tendon. Unfortunately, data on soft tissue graft outcomes and knee stability is lacking. Significant soft tissue graft variability provides the rationale for the original soft tissue graft selection. Unfortunately, lack of data on postoperative knee functionality has hampered comparisons on soft tissue grafts. With the available data, and in cases where preserving the hamstring is the goal, the PLT may be the most justified choice. Appropriate graft selection should be guided by clinical context as the data on ACL reconstruction with PL and HTC grafts is similar. The study achieved its objectives within the stated limitations. However, long-term postoperative functionality outcomes still require further investigation.

10.7. References

Buerba, R.A., Boden, S.A., Lesniak, B. (2021). Graft selection in contemporary anterior cruciate ligament reconstruction. *JAAOS Global Research & Reviews*, 5(10), e21.

Chaitanya, M.K. (2020). Radiological assesement of femoral and tibial tunnel placement in arthroscopic ACL reconstruction using hamstring tendon graft. Master's Thesis, Rajiv Gandhi University of Health Sciences.

Chona, D., Eriksson, K., Young, S.W., Denti, M., Sancheti, P.K., Safran, M., Sherman, S. (2021). Return to sport following anterior cruciate ligament reconstruction: The argument for a multimodal approach to optimise decision-making: Current concepts. *Journal of ISAKOS*, 6(6), 344–348.

D'Ambrosi, R., Giorgino, R., Corona, K., Jaykumar, T., Mariani, I., Ursino, N., Mangiavini, L., Vaishya, R. (2022). Hamstring tendon autografts and allografts show comparable clinical outcomes and knee stability after anterior cruciate ligament reconstruction in patients over fifty years old with no signs of osteoarthritis progression. *International Orthopaedics*, 46(9), 2029–2039.

Ferraz, M.P. (2023). Bone grafts in dental medicine: An overview of autografts, allografts and synthetic materials. *Materials*, 16(11), 4117.

Getgood, A., Hewison, C., Bryant, D., Litchfield, R., Heard, M., Buchko, G., Hiemstra, L.A., Willits, K.R., Firth, A., MacDonald, P. (2020). Stability study group. No difference in functional outcomes when lateral extra-articular tenodesis is added to anterior cruciate ligament reconstruction in young active patients: The stability study. *Arthroscopy: The Journal of Arthroscopic & Related Surgery*, 36(6), 1690–1701.

He, J., Tang, Q., Ernst, S., Linde, M.A., Smolinski, P., Wu, S., Fu, F. (2021). Peroneus longus tendon autograft has functional outcomes comparable to hamstring tendon autograft for anterior cruciate ligament reconstruction: A systematic review and meta-analysis. *Knee Surgery, Sports Traumatology, Arthroscopy*, 29(9), 2869–2879.

de Jong, J., Cutcutache, I., Page, M., Elmoufti, S., Dilley, C., Fröhlich, H., Armstrong, M. (2021). Towards realizing the vision of precision medicine: AI based prediction of clinical drug response. *Brain*, 144(6), 1738–1750.

Khan, A.A., Ahmad, A., Yunus, M.F., Samad, A. (2023). Knee problems and possible support for rehabilitation – A review. *International Journal of Forensic Engineering and Management*, 1(3), 242–262.

Kumar, A., Batta, P., Rathore, P.S., Ahuja, S. (2025). Secure healthcare data sharing and attack detection framework using radial basis neural network. *Scientific Reports*, 15(1), 15432.

Kunze, K.N., Moran, J., Polce, E.M., Pareek, A., Strickland, S.M., Williams, III R.J. (2023). Lower donor site morbidity with hamstring and quadriceps tendon autograft compared with bone-patellar tendon-bone autograft after anterior cruciate ligament reconstruction: A systematic review and network meta-analysis of randomized controlled trials. *Knee Surgery, Sports Traumatology, Arthroscopy*, 31(8), 3339–3352.

Leung, A., DeSandis, B., O'Brien, L., Hammoud, S., Zarzycki, R. (2023). Postoperative considerations based on graft type after anterior cruciate ligament reconstruction a narrative review. *Annals of Joint*, 8, 26.

Lisacek-Kiosoglous, A.B., Powling, A.S., Fontalis, A., Gabr, A., Mazomenos, E., Haddad, F.S. (2023). Artificial intelligence in orthopaedic surgery: Exploring its applications, limitations, and future direction. *Bone & Joint Research*, 12(7), 447–454.

Magnitskaya, N., Mouton, C., Gokeler, A., Nuehrenboerger, C., Pape, D., Seil, R. (2020). Younger age and hamstring tendon graft are associated with higher IKDC 2000 and KOOS scores during the first year after ACL reconstruction. *Knee Surgery, Sports Traumatology, Arthroscopy*, 28(3), 823–832.

Paget, L.D., Sierevelt, I.N., Tol, J.L., Kerkhoffs, G.M., Reurink, G. (2023). The completely patient-reported version of the American Orthopaedic Foot and Ankle Society (AOFAS) score: A valid and reliable measurement for ankle osteoarthritis. *Journal of ISAKOS*, 8(5), 345–351.

Punnoose, D.J., Varghese, J., Theruvil, B., Thomas, A.B. (2024). Peroneus longus tendon autografts have better graft diameter, less morbidity, and enhanced muscle recuperation than hamstring tendon in ACL reconstruction. *Indian Journal of Orthopaedics*, 58(7), 979–986.

Reina, A.E., Sánchez, T.R., Dalla Rosa, J., Sánchez, L.T., Martín, T.B., Arbeloa, L., Serres, J.C., Fernández, G.H., Merinero, R.C., González-García, D. (2021). Diagnosis and management of injuries of the anterior cruciate ligament in skeletally immature patients. A narrative review. *Revista Española de Artroscopia y Cirugía Articular*, 28(2), 111–127.

Rhatomy, S., Abadi, M.B., Setyawan, R., Asikin, A.I., Soekarno, N.R., Imelda, L.G., Budhiparama, N.C. (2021a). Posterior cruciate ligament reconstruction with peroneus longus tendon versus hamstring tendon: A comparison of functional outcome and donor site morbidity. *Knee Surgery, Sports Traumatology, Arthroscopy*, 29(4), 1045–1051.

Rhatomy, S., Chaniago, H., Rasyid, F.A., Phatama, K.Y. (2021b). Comparing the stiffness of peroneus longus tendon versus hamstrings in anterior cruciate ligament reconstruction: A biomechanical study. *Asian Journal of Sports Medicine*, 12(4), e110160.

Rovere, G., Stramazzo, L., Romeo, M., D'Arienzo, A., Maccauro, G., Camarda, L. (2022). Hamstring graft preparation for ACL reconstruction. *Orthopedic Reviews*, 14(5), 38408.

Runer, A., Suter, A., di Sarsina, T.R., Jucho, L., Gföller, P., Csapo, R., Hoser, C., Fink, C. (2023). Quadriceps tendon autograft for primary anterior cruciate ligament reconstruction show comparable clinical, functional, and patient-reported outcome measures, but lower donor-site morbidity compared with hamstring tendon autograft: A matched-pairs study with a mean follow-up of 6.5 years. *Journal of ISAKOS*, 8(2), 60–67.

Senftl, M., Petek, D., Jacobi, M., Schallberger, A., Spycher, J., Stock, A., Hess, R., Tannast, M. (2022). Occurrence of inadequate ACL healing after dynamic intraligamentary stabilization and functional outcome – A multicentre case series. *European Journal of Orthopaedic Surgery & Traumatology*, 32(7), 1265–1274.

Waly, A.H. and Gawish, H.M. (2022). Comparative study between peroneus longus, semitendinosus tendon, and quadriceps tendon graft for anterior cruciate ligament reconstruction. *The Egyptian Orthopaedic Journal*, 57(2), 109–121.

Zhang, S., Cai, G., Ge, Z. (2024). The efficacy of anterior cruciate ligament reconstruction with peroneus longus tendon and its impact on ankle joint function. *Orthopaedic Surgery*, 16(6), 1317–1326.

Zych, R., Mocanu, D., Bokwa-Dąbrowska, K., Dziedzic, D., Szaro, P. (2025). Height and weight predict cross-sectional area of the peroneus brevis and longus tendons: Magnetic resonance imaging-based analysis of 164 adults. *Journal of Experimental Orthopaedics*, 12(4), e70492.

List of Authors

Syed Nadeem AHAMED
Department of Orthopedics
Krishna Institute of Medical Sciences
Krishna Vishwa Vidyapeeth
"Deemed to be University"
Taluka-Karad
India

Priya BATTA
Amity School of Engineering and Technology
Amity University Punjab
Mohali
India

Viradraj Shrinivas DESHMUKH
Department of Orthopedics
Krishna Institute of Medical Sciences
Krishna Vishwa Vidyapeeth
"Deemed to be University"
Taluka-Karad
India

Nikhil DUDHANI
Department of Orthopedics
Krishna Institute of Medical Sciences
Krishna Vishwa Vidyapeeth
"Deemed to be University"
Taluka-Karad
India

Nishant GAONKAR
Department of Orthopedics
Krishna Institute of Medical Sciences
Krishna Vishwa Vidyapeeth
"Deemed to be University"
Taluka-Karad
India

Anshuraj JAGDALE
Department of Orthopedics
Krishna Institute of Medical Sciences
Krishna Vishwa Vidyapeeth
"Deemed to be University"
Taluka-Karad
India

Jineshwar S. KAPALE
Department of Orthopedics
Krishna Institute of Medical Sciences
Krishna Vishwa Vidyapeeth "Deemed to be University"
Taluka-Karad
India

Pradeep N. KULKARNI
Department of Orthopedics
Krishna Institute of Medical Sciences
Krishna Vishwa Vidyapeeth "Deemed to be University"
Taluka-Karad
India

Abhishek KUMAR
Computer Science and Engineering Department
Chandigarh University
Mohali
India

Mrunal PATEL
Department of Orthopedics
Krishna Institute of Medical Sciences
Krishna Vishwa Vidyapeeth "Deemed to be University"
Taluka-Karad
India

Rutul D. PATEL
Department of Orthopedics
Krishna Institute of Medical Sciences
Krishna Vishwa Vidyapeeth "Deemed to be University"
Taluka-Karad
India

Nitin S. PATIL
Department of Orthopedics
Krishna Institute of Medical Sciences
Krishna Vishwa Vidyapeeth "Deemed to be University"
Taluka-Karad
India

Paresh V. PATIL
Department of Orthopedics
Krishna Institute of Medical Sciences
Krishna Vishwa Vidyapeeth "Deemed to be University"
Taluka-Karad
India

Chintalapuri Pranay Bhargav REDDY
Department of Orthopedics
Krishna Institute of Medical Sciences
Krishna Vishwa Vidyapeeth "Deemed to be University"
Taluka-Karad
India

Vikash A. SATRE
Department of Orthopedics
Krishna Institute of Medical Sciences
Krishna Vishwa Vidyapeeth
"Deemed to be University"
Taluka-Karad
India

Nidhi Vipul SHAH
Department of Orthopedics
Krishna Institute of Medical Sciences
Krishna Vishwa Vidyapeeth
"Deemed to be University"
Taluka-Karad
India

Abhishek SHARMA
Department of Orthopedics
Krishna Institute of Medical Sciences
Krishna Vishwa Vidyapeeth
"Deemed to be University"
Taluka-Karad
India

Manthena Ramakrishna Vittal VERMA
Department of Orthopedics
Krishna Institute of Medical Sciences
Krishna Vishwa Vidyapeeth
"Deemed to be University"
Taluka-Karad
India

Index

I, L

M, N, O

P, R

S, T

V, Z

Other titles from

iSTE

in

Computer Engineering

2026

BHAMBRI Pankaj, DUTTA Pushan Kumar, KHAN Mudassir, STAROSTKA-PATYK Marta
Next-Gen Supply Chains: AI, Automation, and Sustainability in a Disrupted World

DARCHE Philippe
Computer Memories 1: Core Concepts
Computer Memories 2: Static Random-Access Memory

KUMAR Abhishek, BATTA Priya, AHUJA Sachin, RATHORE Pramod Singh
AI-driven Innovations in Physiotherapy and Oncology 3

KUMAR Abhishek, BATTA Priya, ANANTH J.P.
AI-driven Healthcare Innovations: Applications in Neurology and Medicine

MACHADO Carolina, DAVIM J. Paulo
Artificial Intelligence Technologies in Management and Engineering

MAHOUT Vincent, ROCACHER Thierry, AURIOL Guillaume
Programming of Embedded Systems: Applications to SM32F10x μControllers

2025

CHIKH Azeddine
Systemic Approach to Categorizing and Modeling Requirements

KUMAR Abhishek, BATTA Priya, AHUJA Sachin,
RATHORE Pramod Singh
AI-driven Innovations in Physiotherapy and Oncology 1
AI-driven Innovations in Physiotherapy and Oncology 2

TANEJA Ashu, KUMAR Abhishek, LIMKAR Suresh Vishnudas,
OUAISSA Mariya, OUAISSA Mariyam
Driving Innovation through AI and Digital Twin for 6G Powered Sustainable Ultra Smart Cities

TANEJA Ashu, KUMAR Abhishek, LIMKAR Suresh Vishnudas,
OUAISSA Mariya, OUAISSA Mariyam
6G Urban Innovation: AI and Digital Twin for Next-Gen Sustainable Cities

2024

CHAKRABORTY Rajdeep, GHOSH Anupam, KUMAR MANDAL Jyotsna,
CHOUDHURY Tanupriya, CHATTERJEE Prasenjit
Smart Edge Computing: An Operation Research Perspective
(International Perspectives in Decision Analytics and Operations Research Set – Volume 2)

HOMÈS Bernard
Fundamentals of Software Testing (2nd edition, revised and updated)

JERBI Abdessalem
Discrete-Event Simulation: Concepts and Production in Arena

PRADHAN Devasis, KUMAR SAHU Prasanna, MYO TUN Hla,
CHATTERJEE Prasenjit
Artificial and Cognitive Computing for Sustainable Healthcare Systems in Smart Cities
(International Perspectives in Decision Analytics and Operations Research Set – Volume 3)

2023

CHOUDHURY Tanupriya, KHANNA Abhirup, CHATTERJEE Prasenjit, UM Jung-Sup, BHATTACHARYA Abhishek
Blockchain Applications in Healthcare: Innovations and Practices (International Perspectives in Decision Analytics and Operations Research Set – Volume 1)

PAI G A Vijayalakshmi
A Textbook of Data Structures and Algorithms 1: Mastering Linear Data Structures
A Textbook of Data Structures and Algorithms 2: Mastering Nonlinear Data Structures
A Textbook of Data Structures and Algorithms 3: Mastering Advanced Data Structures and Algorithm Design Strategies

2022

HOMÈS Bernard
Advanced Testing of Systems-of-Systems 1: Theoretical Aspects
Advanced Testing of Systems-of-Systems 2: Practical Aspects

MEHTA Shikha, TIWARI Sanju, SIARRY Patrick, JABBAR M.A.
Tools, Languages, Methodologies for Representing Semantics on the Web of Things

SIDHOM Sahbi, KADDOUR Amira
Systems and Uses of Digital Sciences for Knowledge Organization (Digital Tools and Uses Set – Volume 9)

ZAIDOUN Ameur Salem
Computer Science Security: Concepts and Tools

2021

DARCHE Philippe
Microprocessor 4: Core Concepts – Software Aspects
Microprocessor 5: Software and Hardware Aspects of Development, Debugging and Testing – The Microcomputer

DELHAYE Jean-Loïc
Inside the World of Computing: Technologies, Uses, Challenges

HARDIN Thérèse, JAUME Mathieu, PESSAUX François,
VIGUIÉ DONZEAU-GOUGE Véronique
Concepts and Semantics of Programming Languages 1: A Semantical Approach with OCaml and Python
Concepts and Semantics of Programming Languages 2: Modular and Object-oriented Constructs with OCaml, Python, C++, Ada and Java

MKADMI Abderrazak
Archives in The Digital Age: Preservation and the Right to be Forgotten (Digital Tools and Uses Set – Volume 8)

TOKLU Yusuf Cengiz, BEKDAŞ Gebrail, NIGDELI Sinan Melih
Metaheuristics for Structural Design and Analysis (Optimization Heuristics Set – Volume 3)

2020

DARCHE Philippe
Microprocessor 1: Prolegomenes – Calculation and Storage Functions – Models of Computation and Computer Architecture
Microprocessor 2: Core Concepts – Communication in a Digital System
Microprocessor 3: Core Concepts – Hardware Aspects

DUVAUT Patrick, DALLOZ Xavier, MENGA David, KOEHL François,
CHRIQUI Vidal, BRILL Joerg
Internet of Augmented Me, I.AM: Empowering Innovation for a New Sustainable Future

LAFFLY Dominique
TORUS 1 – Toward an Open Resource Using Services: Cloud Computing for Environmental Data
TORUS 2 – Toward an Open Resource Using Services: Cloud Computing for Environmental Data
TORUS 3 – Toward an Open Resource Using Services: Cloud Computing for Environmental Data

LAURENT Anne, LAURENT Dominique, MADERA Cédrine
Data Lakes
(Databases and Big Data Set – Volume 2)

OULHADJ Hamouche, DAACHI Boubaker, MENASRI Riad
Metaheuristics for Robotics
(Optimization Heuristics Set – Volume 2)

SADIQUI Ali
Computer Network Security

VENTRE Daniel
Artificial Intelligence, Cybersecurity and Cyber Defense

2019

BESBES Walid, DHOUIB Diala, WASSAN Niaz, MARREKCHI Emna
Solving Transport Problems: Towards Green Logistics

CLERC Maurice
Iterative Optimizers: Difficulty Measures and Benchmarks

GHLALA Riadh
Analytic SQL in SQL Server 2014/2016

TOUNSI Wiem
Cyber-Vigilance and Digital Trust: Cyber Security in the Era of Cloud Computing and IoT

2018

ANDRO Mathieu
Digital Libraries and Crowdsourcing
(Digital Tools and Uses Set – Volume 5)

ARNALDI Bruno, GUITTON Pascal, MOREAU Guillaume
Virtual Reality and Augmented Reality: Myths and Realities

CARDON Alain
Beyond Artificial Intelligence: From Human Consciousness to Artificial Consciousness

HOMAYOUNI S. Mahdi, FONTES Dalila B.M.M.
Metaheuristics for Maritime Operations
(Optimization Heuristics Set – Volume 1)

JEANSOULIN Robert
JavaScript and Open Data

PIVERT Olivier
NoSQL Data Models: Trends and Challenges
(Databases and Big Data Set – Volume 1)

SEDKAOUI Soraya
Data Analytics and Big Data

SALEH Imad, AMMI Mehdi, SZONIECKY Samuel
Challenges of the Internet of Things: Technology, Use, Ethics
(Digital Tools and Uses Set – Volume 7)

SZONIECKY Samuel
Ecosystems Knowledge: Modeling and Analysis Method for Information and Communication
(Digital Tools and Uses Set – Volume 6)

2017

BENMAMMAR Badr
Concurrent, Real-Time and Distributed Programming in Java: Threads, RTSJ and RMI

BOUHAÏ Nasreddine, SALEH Imad
Internet of Things: Evolutions and Innovations
(Digital Tools and Uses Set – Volume 4)

HÉLIODORE Frédéric, NAKIB Amir, ISMAIL Boussaad, OUCHRAA Salma, SCHMITT Laurent
Metaheuristics for Intelligent Electrical Networks
(Metaheuristics Set – Volume 10)

MA Haiping, SIMON Dan
Evolutionary Computation with Biogeography-based Optimization
(Metaheuristics Set – Volume 8)

PÉTROWSKI Alain, BEN-HAMIDA Sana
Evolutionary Algorithms
(Metaheuristics Set – Volume 9)

PAI G A Vijayalakshmi
Metaheuristics for Portfolio Optimization: An Introduction using MATLAB®
(Metaheuristics Set – Volume 11)

REYES-GARCIA Everardo
The Image-Interface: Graphical Supports for Visual Information
(Digital Tools and Uses Set – Volume 3)

REYES-GARCIA Everardo, BOUHAÏ Nasreddine
Designing Interactive Hypermedia Systems
(Digital Tools and Uses Set – Volume 2)

SZONIECKY Samuel, BOUHAÏ Nasreddine
Collective Intelligence and Digital Archives: Towards Knowledge Ecosystems
(Digital Tools and Uses Set – Volume 1)

2016

BLUM Christian, FESTA Paola
Metaheuristics for String Problems in Bio-informatics
(Metaheuristics Set – Volume 6)

DEROUSSI Laurent
Metaheuristics for Logistics
(Metaheuristics Set – Volume 4)

DHAENENS Clarisse, JOURDAN Laetitia
Metaheuristics for Big Data
(Metaheuristics Set – Volume 5)

LABADIE Nacima, PRINS Christian, PRODHON Caroline
Metaheuristics for Vehicle Routing Problems
(Metaheuristics Set – Volume 3)

LEROY Laure
Eyestrain Reduction in Stereoscopy

LUTTON Evelyne, PERROT Nathalie, TONDA Alberto
Evolutionary Algorithms for Food Science and Technology
(Metaheuristics Set – Volume 7)

MAGOULÈS Frédéric, ZHAO Hai-Xiang
Data Mining and Machine Learning in Building Energy Analysis

RIGO Michel
Advanced Graph Theory and Combinatorics

ZELM Martin, DOUMEINGTS Guy, MENDONÇA Joao Pedro
Enterprise Interoperability: in the Digitized and Networked Factory of the Future

2015

BARBIER Franck, RECOUSSINE Jean-Luc
COBOL Software Modernization: From Principles to Implementation with the BLU AGE® Method

CHEN Ken
Performance Evaluation by Simulation and Analysis with Applications to Computer Networks

CLERC Maurice
Guided Randomness in Optimization
(Metaheuristics Set – Volume 1)

DURAND Nicolas, GIANAZZA David, GOTTELAND Jean-Baptiste, ALLIOT Jean-Marc
Metaheuristics for Air Traffic Management
(Metaheuristics Set – Volume 2)

MAGOULÈS Frédéric, ROUX François-Xavier, HOUZEAUX Guillaume
Parallel Scientific Computing

MUNEESAWANG Paisarn, YAMMEN Suchart
Visual Inspection Technology in the Hard Disk Drive Industry

2014

BOULANGER Jean-Louis
Formal Methods Applied to Industrial Complex Systems
Formal Methods Applied to Complex Systems: Implementation of the B Method

EXPOSITO Ernesto, DIOP Codé
Smart SOA Platforms in Cloud Computing Architectures

GARDI Frédéric, BENOIST Thierry, DARLAY Julien, ESTELLON Bertrand, MEGEL Romain
Mathematical Programming Solver based on Local Search

KRICHEN Saoussen, CHAOUACHI Jouhaina
Graph-related Optimization and Decision Support Systems

LARRIEU Nicolas, VARET Antoine
Rapid Prototyping of Software for Avionics Systems: Model-oriented Approaches for Complex Systems Certification

LAURAS Matthieu, ZELM Martin, ARCHIMÈDE Bernard, BÉNABEN Frédérick, DOUMEINGTS Guy
Enterprise Interoperability: Interoperability for Agility, Resilience and Plasticity of Collaborations

OUSSALAH Mourad Chabane
Software Architecture 1
Software Architecture 2

QUESNEL Flavien
Scheduling of Large-scale Virtualized Infrastructures: Toward Cooperative Management

RIGO Michel
Formal Languages, Automata and Numeration Systems 1: Introduction to Combinatorics on Words
Formal Languages, Automata and Numeration Systems 2: Applications to Recognizability and Decidability

SAINT-DIZIER Patrick
Musical Rhetoric: Foundations and Annotation Schemes

TOUATI Sid, DUPONT DE DINECHIN Benoit
Advanced Backend Code Optimization

2013

ANDRÉ Étienne, SOULAT Romain
The Inverse Method: Parametric Verification of Real-time Embedded Systems

BOULANGER Jean-Louis
Safety Management for Software-based Equipment

DELAHAYE Daniel, PUECHMOREL Stéphane
Modeling and Optimization of Air Traffic

FRANCOPOULO Gil
LMF — Lexical Markup Framework

GHEDIRA Khaled
Constraint Satisfaction Problems: CSP Formalisms and Techniques

GOVAERT Gérard, NADIF Mohamed
Co-Clustering: Models, Algorithms and Applications

LANDRAGIN Frédérick
Man–Machine Dialogue: Design and Challenges

LUCAS Laurent, LOSCOS Céline, REMION Yannick
3D Video: Models, From Capture to Diffusion

ROCHANGE Christine, UHRIG Sascha, SAINRAT Pascal
Time-Predictable Architectures

WAHBI Mohamed
Algorithms and Ordering Heuristics for Distributed Constraint Satisfaction Problems

ZELM Martin, VAN SINDEREN Marten, FERRAIRA PIRES Luis, DOUMEINGTS Guy
Enterprise Interoperability: Research and Applications in the Service-oriented Ecosystem

2012

ARBOLEDA Hugo, ROYER Jean-Claude
Model-Driven and Software Product Line Engineering

BLANCHET Gérard, DUPOUY Bertrand
Computer Architecture

BOULANGER Jean-Louis
Industrial Use of Formal Methods: Formal Verification
Formal Methods: Industrial Use from Model to the Code

CALVARY Gaëlle, DELOT Thierry, SÈDES Florence, TIGLI Jean-Yves
Computer Science and Ambient Intelligence

MAHOUT Vincent
Assembly Language Programming: ARM Cortex-M3 2.0: Organization, Innovation and Territory

MARLET Renaud
Program Specialization

SOTO Maria, SEVAUX Marc, ROSSI André, LAURENT Johann
Memory Allocation Problems in Embedded Systems: Optimization Methods

2011

BICHOT Charles-Edmond, SIARRY Patrick
Graph Partitioning

BOULANGER Jean-Louis
Static Analysis of Software: The Abstract Interpretation

CAFERRA Ricardo
Logic for Computer Science and Artificial Intelligence

KORDON Fabrice, HADDAD Serge, PAUTET Laurent, PETRUCCI Laure
Distributed Systems: Design and Algorithms
Models and Analysis in Distributed Systems

LORCA Xavier
Tree-based Graph Partitioning Constraint

RIDHA MAHJOUB A.
Progress in Combinatorial Optimization: ISCO2010

TRUCHET Charlotte, ASSAYAG Gerard
Constraint Programming in Music

VICAT-BLANC Pascale, GOGLIN Brice, GUILLIER Romaric,
SOUDAN Sébastien
Computing Networks: From Cluster to Cloud Computing

2010

AUBRUN Christophe, SIMON Daniel, SONG Ye-Qiong
Co-design Approaches for Dependable Networked Control Systems

AUDIBERT Pierre
Mathematics for Informatics and Computer Science

BABAU Jean-Philippe, BLAY-FORNARINO Mireille, CHAMPEAU Joël,
ROBERT Sylvain, SABETTA Antonino
Model Driven Engineering for Distributed Real-Time Systems: MARTE Modeling, Model Transformations and their Usages

BOULANGER Jean-Louis
Safety of Computer Architectures

SIGAUD Olivier, BUFFET Olivier
Markov Decision Processes in Artificial Intelligence

MONMARCHÉ Nicolas, GUINAND Frédérick, SIARRY Patrick
Artificial Ants

SOLNON Christine
Ant Colony Optimization and Constraint Programming

2009

FOURNIER Jean-Claude
Graph Theory and Applications: with exercises and problems

GUÉDON Jeanpierre
The Mojette Transform: theory and applications

JARD Claude, ROUX Olivier H.
Communicating Embedded Systems: Software and Design

LECOUTRE Christophe
Constraint Networks: Techniques and Algorithms

2008

BANÂTRE Michel, MARRON Pedro Jose, OLLERO Anibal, WOLITZ Adam
Cooperating Embedded Systems and Wireless Sensor Networks

MERZ Stephan, NAVET Nicolas
Modeling and Verification of Real-time Systems: Formalisms and Software Tools

PASCHOS Vangelis Th.
Combinatorial Optimization and Theoretical Computer Science: Interfaces and Perspectives

WALDNER Jean-Baptiste
Nanocomputers and Swarm Intelligence

2007

BENHAMOU Frédéric, JUSSIEN Narendra, O'SULLIVAN Barry
Trends in Constraint Programming

JUSSIEN Narendra
A to Z of Sudoku

2006

BABAU Jean-Philippe, CHAMPEAU Joël, GÉRARD Sébastien
From MDD Concepts to Experiments and Illustrations – DRES 2006

HABRIAS Henri, FRAPPIER Marc
Software Specification Methods: An Overview Using a Case Study

MURAT Cécile, PASCHOS Vangelis Th.
Probabilistic Combinatorial Optimization on Graphs

PANETTO Hervé, BOUDJLIDA Nacer
Interoperability for Enterprise Software and Applications: Proceedings of the Workshops and the Doctorial Symposium of the Second IFAC/IFIP I-ESA International Conference: EI2N, WSI, IS-TSPQ 2006

2005

GÉRARD Sébastien, BABAU Jean-Philippe, CHAMPEAU Joël
Model Driven Engineering for Distributed Real Time Embedded Systems

PANETTO Hervé
Interoperability of Enterprise Software and Applications: Workshops of the INTEROP-ESA 2005 International Conference (EI2N, WSI, ISIDI and IEHENA 2005)

Printed and bound by CPI Group (UK) Ltd, Croydon, CR0 4YY
16/09/2026
14963201-0002